CARIBBEAN FAMILY LIFE
· A PRACTICAL GUIDE ·
ELAINE ROBERTSON

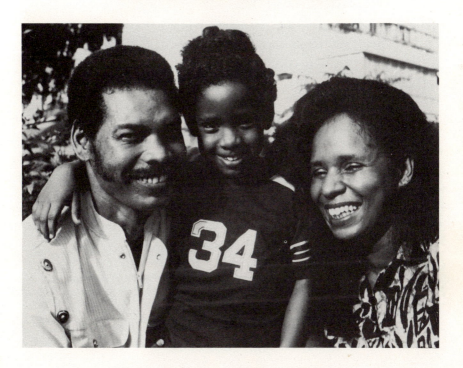

CAMBRIDGE UNIVERSITY PRESS
Cambridge
New York   New Rochelle
Melbourne   Sydney

Elaine Robertson

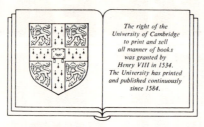

*The right of the
University of Cambridge
to print and sell
all manner of books
was granted by
Henry VIII in 1534.
The University has printed
and published continuously
since 1584.*

Published by the Press Syndicate of the University of Cambridge
The Pitt Building, Trumpington Street, Cambridge CB2 1RP
32 East 57th Street, New York, NY 10022, USA
10 Stamford Road, Oakleigh, Melbourne 3166, Australia

© Cambridge University Press 1987

First published 1987

Printed in Great Britain by Scotprint, Musselburgh, Scotland

ISBN 0 521 31944 7

Acknowledgements

First and foremost, the author would like to say thank you to all the young people with whom she has had contact on her child-care courses in Trinidad and London. Author – and publisher – would also like to thank Mrs Pauline Murphy, Nursing Sister, Kingston School of Nursing, and Mrs Angela Senior, Senior Nurse Tutor, Continuing Education, Leeds Eastern Health Authority, for their helpful advice and assistance.

Author and publisher gratefully acknowledge the following for permission to reproduce illustrations in this book: the Bureau of Health Education, Ministry of Health and Environmental Control, Kingston, Jamaica, WI, for the various extracts from their health education leaflets; © Geoff Jones for the biological diagrams on pages 33, 34, 37, 38, 41, and 42; Farley Health Products Ltd for the photographs on pages 40, 76, 80, and 94; Antony Rose for the photograph on page 4; David Runnacles for the photographs on pages 87–9 and 104; Neil Sutton for line illustrations on pages 46, 103–6, 111, and 132–3; Robert Small for the photograph on page 175.

All other line illustrations specially commissioned from Pauline Henry. All other photographs specially commissioned from Harold Oxley.

We would also like to thank all the parents and children who have allowed their photographs to be used.

Contents

To parents, parents-to-be and their children   page 5

PART ONE: The family   7
Introduction   7
  1 Family patterns   11
  2 Becoming a parent   21

PART TWO: How human life begins   31
  3 Where do babies come from?   31
  4 Pre-natal development   41
  5 Pregnancy   51
  6 Birth of a baby   63

PART THREE: The early years   73
  7 The physical care of the baby   73
  8 Coping with a new baby   95
  9 The importance of the first years   101
  10 Caring for the toddler   115
  11 The value of play   129
  12 The handicapped child   139
  13 Illness and accidents   145
  14 The toddler goes to nursery school   163
  15 Nursery school to infant school   167

Index   175

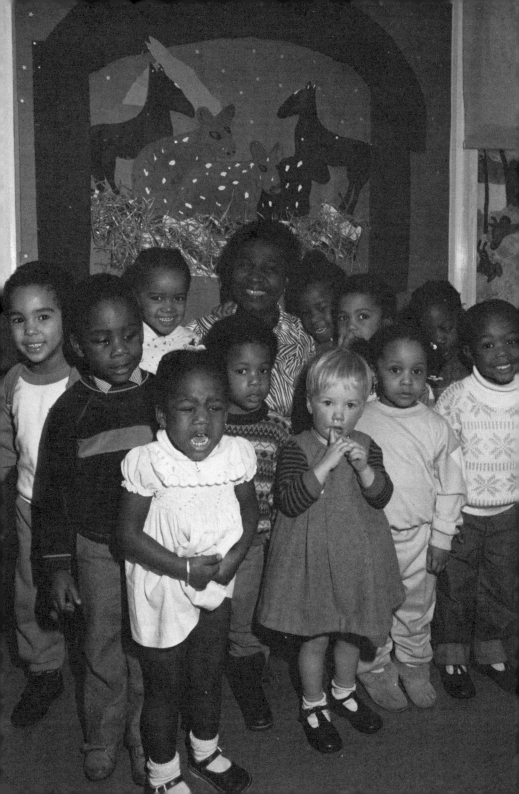

To parents, parents-to-be and their children

During several years of organising and teaching child-care courses in Trinidad, I met and talked with many young people, both boys and girls, who were keenly interested in learning 'the facts of life' as accurately as possible.

There were those who, growing up in families with younger brothers and sisters, and noticing the changes in their mothers' bodies during pregnancy, asked why this was so. Their experiences of their mothers' reactions varied. Some remembered being simply told that a baby brother or sister was there, and were even allowed to feel the movements of the baby. This was exciting and strange, but never was an explanation given of how the baby came to be there. Others were firmly told not to ask rude questions nor be concerned with 'big people's business'. These answers left them curious and eager to find out more, and as they grew older they obtained bits of information from friends who were not always 'too sure'.

The disadvantage of learning from friends was that very often some of the information was inaccurate, and how the reproductory system of the body worked was not fully understood; some young people who engaged in sexual intercourse found themselves, to their surprise, 'in the family way'. In most cases their school careers ended, much to the disappointment and anger of their parents.

This book aims to help you understand the importance of the family, how human life begins, and discusses how the child develops during its early years. I hope that the knowledge gained will be useful to many people in the Caribbean, either in their present family, or when they eventually have children of their own, or in a career connected with child care.

E E Robertson.

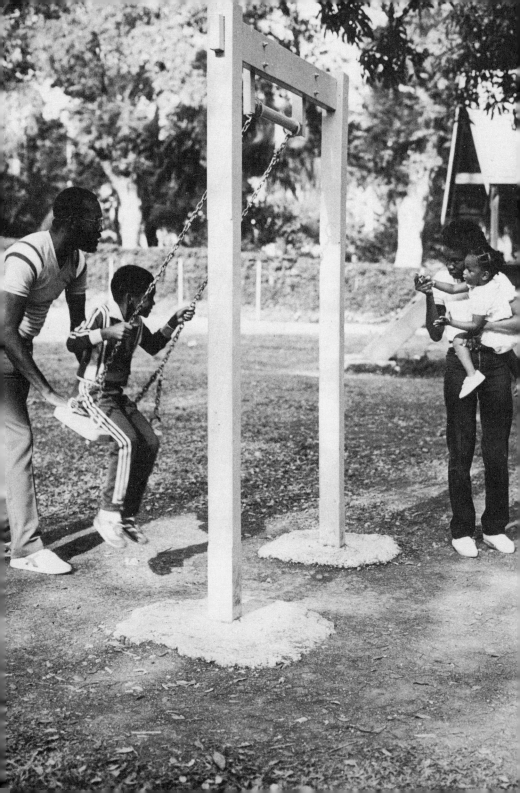

PART ONE: THE FAMILY

Introduction

Human beings generally value the company of others and choose to live together in large or small groups. When a group of people voluntarily occupy the same living accommodation and share at least one meal a day, this group is defined as a household. The household usually consists of a family unit – a couple or a single parent with child or children. But, in the Caribbean, the household can consist of the family unit and other relatives, or others who are not blood relations but who are accepted and treated as if they are. On the other hand, not all the members of the family unit necessarily live in the household; often it is the father who is non-resident, but there are instances where it may be the mother. The cause of their absence may be migration to the town or to an overseas country in search of employment

One important aspect of family life which is universally accepted is that children need to be cared for and protected. The family is expected to provide the basic necessities of life: shelter, food, clothing, and, where necessary, warmth. The family also provides for the emotional needs of the child, giving love, affection and security, which are all necessary for the development of the child's basic trust. This will help him or her to form relationships with others at a later stage and provide the basis for understanding the customs of the society in which the family lives.

There are times when, for a number of reasons, some families are unable to make the provisions listed above, then either relatives, or government or voluntary agencies assume responsibility for the care of the children. Most countries pay special attention to keeping the family together, realising that the hope of the society's future rests with young people.

THE GENERATION GAP

It is natural for differences to exist between generations within a family. Some families have no difficulty in bridging the gap because they are able to communicate and discuss the pros and cons of certain customs which may have been followed within that particular household for many years. Changing conditions in the outer world may suggest and demand the need for some adaptations to be made, and the older members in those families try to understand and accept the need for change. Conflict occurs when the elders within a family are rigid, resist change and tend to remind everyone: 'In my day, that would not be allowed.' Often, the younger members of the family may not be permitted to state their point of view. On the other hand, the younger members may be intolerant and expect the elders to change to their way of thinking. In these instances the generation gap widens, causing everyone to be uncomfortable and unhappy. This is unfortunate, for many elderly people possess great wisdom and experience which can be shared with the young.

DIFFERENCES

Some families discourage their young children from mixing with others who are considered different. The difference may be in social position or economic status among people like themselves, or those who practise different religions or are of a different race or skin colour. Not mixing with others can lead to a very narrow, prejudiced view of people different from oneself. Those parents who appreciate differences are able to help their young children to understand the multi-racial and multi-cultural nature of the world. Because so many different races have settled in the Caribbean islands, the population is a rich and varied mixture. In some families there are members who may be very different in skin colour, but they learn to accept and relate to one another.

FAMILY FINANCES

Careful planning and budgeting help in making the best use of money which may come from wages or salaries earned by one or other parent, or by both. Where there are grown-up offspring still living in the home, they also contribute some of their earnings. In some countries governments provide grants of money for adults who are unemployed. They may also provide pensions for the elderly. Help may be given to families in the form of assistance with fares for transport of the elderly and blind, or with children's schoolbooks, school uniforms and school lunches.

Each family has to think carefully how it can survive best with the amount of money it controls, and not involve itself in debt with purchases which it cannot afford in order to keep up with the family next door. Young children will ask parents for articles which they see in shops or in the homes of their friends. For many parents this can be very difficult, but young children are quite capable of understanding an explanation about the need to wait and save in order to buy the desired item. When the family enjoys a warm and close relationship, it is much easier for the child to accept the parents' decision.

HAPPY FAMILIES

Some families succeed in living happily together. They are not necessarily rich, but the members are loving and caring towards one another. They talk frankly, spend time in one another's company, and share joys and sorrows. The various talents and abilities of individuals are used for the benefit of all. Whilst the head of the family plays a large part in creating the atmosphere of the home, much depends on the co-operation of every member of the family.

There are those families whose happiness is based on strong religious beliefs which influence their way of life. The various peoples of the Caribbean observe different religious practices. These include: Christians, both in the established churches and the non-conformist churches; Muslims and Hindus; and many who, while they do not believe in formal religion, live by moral codes and pass these on to their children. One of these codes often instilled in children is 'Do unto others as you would have done unto you.' Responsible adults in the family help children to respect and show tolerance to those who possess different beliefs, and to realise that it is possible to coexist in peace and harmony.

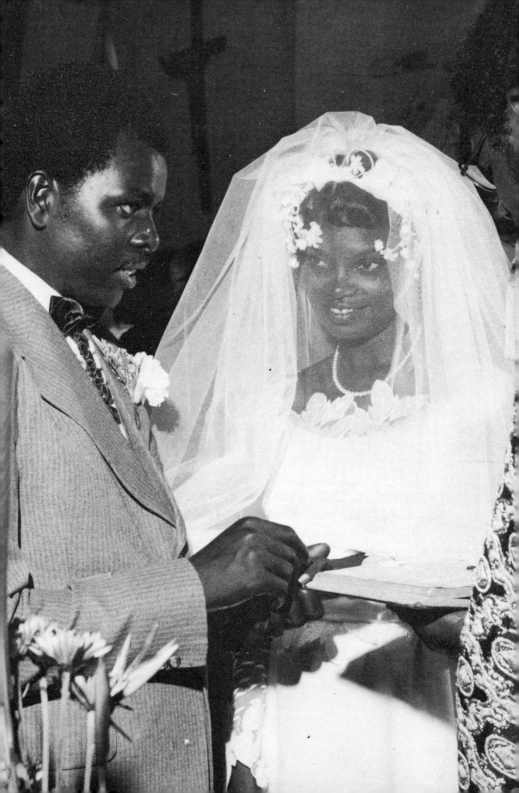

1 Family patterns

Look around at the families you know and they will probably fall into one of the following three patterns:
the **extended** family – grandparents, other relatives, parents and their children
the **nuclear** family – father, mother and their children
the **single** or **one-parent** family – a mother **or** father and children.

Since each pattern of family depends initially on a couple getting together, let us first look at some of the ways this is done.

CHOOSING A PARTNER

In some instances boys and girls growing up in the same village or street of a town may be attracted to each other from an early age and become 'childhood sweethearts'. If their parents consent, they may marry at an early age or they may decide to wait until they are legally able to do so. The minimum age at which a legal marriage can be contracted varies from 12 to 16 in the various Caribbean countries. During the early part of the present century, among the Afro-Caribbean population, village life was very closely knit and women were expected to remain in the home. Girls were taught 'needling', embroidery, crochet, washing and cooking – and prior to marriage they were treated as children, remaining under the constant supervision of adults.

Many older people recall the practice of the young man 'writing home' to the young woman's parents asking permission to marry her. If the parents did not approve of him the letter was returned and the girl was forbidden to see him, but if the young man was accepted, the families exchanged visits and they discussed how long the couple would remain engaged before marrying. During this time the young man would work and save enough money to build or buy a house, and the young woman prepared her 'bottom drawer' with hand-made and embroidered articles such as pillowcases, towels, tablecloths and items of clothing. This was called the 'trousseau'. The young man visited his fiancée's home, but the couple always spoke to each other in the presence of her parents. When they went out they were accompanied by a member of the family. Neither was expected to be seen alone with someone of the opposite sex. Legally, an engagement was, and still is, considered as a contract and if it is broken by one or the other, court action may be taken for 'breach of promise'. The court has the power to make the offender pay any expenses the other may have had in preparation for the wedding. The embarrassment of publicity prevents some people from going to court if an engagement is broken off, but in some islands cases have been successfully contested, usually by the girl's parents.

Nowadays in the Caribbean there is a mixture of formal engagements and couples choosing each other from among those they meet at work or at college or university, or even in their travels abroad.

Among some families of East Indian origin living in the Caribbean, the tradition of parents selecting partners for their children is still practised. In the larger islands, the young people may never have met, but in recent times, since boys and girls are often educated together, there is the opportunity for them to get to know each other. Even if this is so, the older family members of one group make a formal approach to the other family and discuss marriage plans, provided the young man or woman is acceptable to the family. This would depend on whether he or she is of the same religion, social position, or educational or economic level.

Usually, when a couple decide to marry, the wedding is a large social gathering of relatives and friends and the arrangements are the responsibility of the bride's parents. But there are many couples who do not follow the formality of an engagement and live together before deciding to marry. Very often at a later stage they marry in a similar, elaborate fashion.

MARRIAGE

Marriage is the legal union between a man and a woman, making them husband and wife. It is a serious decision taken by the couple who feel that they love, trust and respect each other to the extent that they promise to live together for the rest of their lives; if and when children are born to them, together they protect and care for them in a secure and loving atmosphere in the home. If one or other of the partners continues the same style of life as when single, or is selfish to the extent that his or her way must be accepted at all times, the marriage runs the risk of breaking up. In successful marriages partners give and take, and make allowances for each other's faults. They communicate with each other and share joy and sorrow; they help each other, and are companions to each other.

The husband is obliged by law to maintain (provide financially for) his family. Among most people living in the Caribbean it is usual for the man's name to become the family name. The wife stops using her surname and the children are all given the father's surname. For example, Mr George Evans marries Miss Edith Green, and they are known as Mr and Mrs George Evans; professionally the wife may be referred to as Mrs Edith Evans. In recent times, however, a growing number of professional women have kept their own surnames at work: Edith Green.

The father is legally responsible for the children until they 'come of age'. The expression means being recognised by the law of the country as an adult with the right to vote, and free to marry without parents' consent. In the UK and many of the Commonwealth Caribbean islands, twenty-one was the age, but it has now been lowered to eighteen. This event is marked in some families by entertaining relatives and friends at a party. Formerly there used to be the symbolic presentation of a key to the young man or woman as a sign that he or she was now capable of accepting responsibility for themselves. Today having one's own key is not so significant since many children of working parents are given keys at an early age and are expected to look after themselves if they return home from school before their parents.

The marriage ceremony

In order for a marriage to be legally recognised, there are certain requirements laid down by law. The age requirements have already been mentioned. Another requirement is that the ceremony must be performed by a priest or lay person who is licensed. It can take place in religious buildings such as cathedrals, churches, temples, mosques, synagogues; or in civic buildings such as town halls, community centres; or in private homes, tents or gardens. Indeed, a marriage may take place wherever the couple chooses. Some couples have chosen to be married in aeroplanes high in the

THE FAMILY

sky, or under water in submarines; some at dawn, some at dusk, depending on how unusual and romantic they wish the occasion to be. In Trinidad and Tobago many Hindu marriages were performed in temporary extensions to houses; the extension was usually made of bamboo and the custom was described as 'marrying under bamboo'. It was not until 1946 that these marriages were considered legal. Some couples exchange rings. In some marriages, only the woman receives a ring from the bridegroom. A certificate of marriage is signed by the couple in front of not less than two witnesses. The marriage is registered and kept in the records of the country.

COMMON LAW UNION

A couple may decide to live together without marrying. Such a union is called a 'common law' union. The man takes care of the family as in a legal marriage, but the mother is legally responsible for the children, who usually carry her surname. In some instances, if the father's name is included on the children's birth certificates, they are entitled to carry his name.

In the Caribbean, many couples live in common law union in stable family homes. But some women may feel very insecure for themselves and their children when the relationship is not working, since the man is under no legal obligation to support her or the children if he leaves. The mother can take the matter to court, and the court may order payment of maintenance by the father, but sometimes the amount is very small. Another disadvantage in common law union is that the partners do not inherit property automatically, as a married person would, when either partner dies intestate (without making a will). The relatives of the common law partner may claim the property if they wish. In some of the islands the law has been changed recently in order to make it easier for children born out of wedlock to inherit property from their fathers where paternity has been established.

DIVORCE

A couple may find themselves unable to live together without serious disagreements on almost every matter in the home. Quarrels and fights are frequent, or they refuse to speak to each other, very often using older children as messengers, for example, 'Tell your mother . . .' or 'Tell your father I'm going out.' The atmosphere in the home then becomes very strained and unpleasant.

Some couples who are reluctant to part may try to discuss their problems with their priest, or selected relatives or friends; if these are unable to help they may seek the help of social workers or marriage guidance counsellors. When all these efforts fail, one or other partner may decide to petition the court for a divorce on the grounds that the marriage has broken down and cannot be repaired.

Sometimes one or other partner deserts the home. If there is no contact between the couple for a certain length of time laid down by law, the partner who has been left may make the petition to the court for the divorce. In most countries of the Commonwealth Caribbean a petition cannot be presented to the court until three years of the marriage have passed.

Most religions regard marriage as binding for life, but if all the circumstances of the couple are carefully considered, and if parting would be in their best interests and that of the children, divorce is allowed. Nevertheless, no matter what the reasons are, divorce can be distressing to the couple and their children, and to relatives. Many parents experience difficulty in explaining divorce to their children, who can be bewildered and confused when one parent leaves home.

Generally it is helpful if children are not encouraged to take sides. Social workers who are brought in to help the family hope that parents are able to maintain the good relationships they may have had with their children before the divorce, but if a parent has maltreated the children, the court decides with whom they will live, and when, where, and for how long the offending parent may see them.

THE EXTENDED FAMILY

In this type of family a young man or woman marries or establishes a common law union and continues to live in the family home. If the couple have children, the first parents become grandparents and the brothers and sisters become uncles and aunts to the couple's children. The extended family group may all live in one house, or in separate houses in the same yard, or in houses next to each other on the same street. In many countries, particularly

THE FAMILY

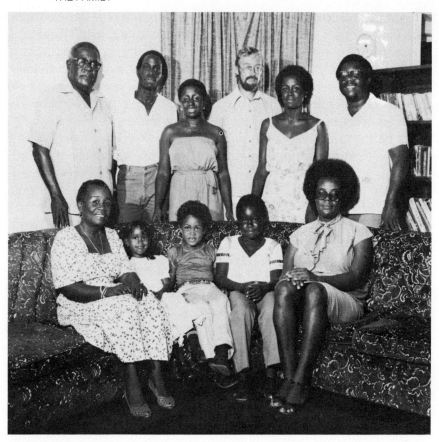

The extended family

where the main occupation of the people is agriculture, the extended family is important as a source of labour. Some families also run their businesses with the help of members of the extended family.

In the extended family there are usually other family members – such as the grandmother – to assist in the care of the young children. If the parents go out to work or leave the home for any other reason, the children's routine is not disrupted. This does not mean that a young child does not miss its parents, but the familiar home environment and the familiar faces help to make the feeling of loss bearable.

Many grandparents can be a source of comfort to children in the family and play an important part in their upbringing. On the other hand, one or other of the grandparents, and in many instances grandmother, may be very critical of the young wife or husband and disagree with their method of child-rearing. Such a situation can be very confusing for the children and the whole family. Sometimes there may be overcrowding in the home and there is very little privacy for anyone. This can lead to frustration and bad temper and frequent bickering; but if an extended family lives in a household with sufficient space in which everyone is comfortable, children grow up learning to live with a number of people of different temperaments, and this is excellent preparation for living in a wider community.

THE NUCLEAR FAMILY

When a man and woman live in their own home with their children, this family group is known as a nuclear family. The nuclear family may live in the same house, yard or compound as the parents of one or both partners, or may move away to be near the husband's place of work or the children's school, or they may emigrate to another country. In any event, the couple are independent of their own parents and bring up their children in the way they think is best. Their parents and other relatives may visit frequently or only on special occasions such as birthdays.

The nuclear family that lives far away from relatives, in their own country or abroad, can be very isolated. Nowadays it is common for both parents to work outside the home and they either depend on domestic helpers to look after the children, or take them to day nurseries where these are available. Sometimes, as the children grow older they are left more and more on their own. Some boys and girls do not seem to mind this arrangement, but others appear to be very lonely and disappointed at not having anyone to welcome them home and to share the day's experiences. It is not much fun taking home a picture which is thought to be beautiful, or a book full of correct sums, if there is no one to admire or praise the achievement. Some parents are too tired when they get home in the evenings to take any notice, or the children are too sleepy to try to interest them. In these cases, watching television can be a favourite pastime for many, but children who are physically active may join others in the street or playground. This is a crucial time when the more adventurous may get into trouble by breaking the law. Fortunately, there are organisations such as the Scout and Girl Guide Movements, Junior Red Cross, St John's Ambulance Brigade, Pathfinders, dance or drama clubs, junior steel bands and the like, where a lot of free time may be spent. Unfortunately, there are some parents who cannot afford the subscriptions for their children to join these organisations; these are the children who are in great danger of becoming delinquent. Parents who work need to think carefully about making arrangements for the supervision of their children after school and during the holidays.

THE ONE-PARENT FAMILY

For reasons such as death, desertion, prolonged illness in hospital, separation or divorce, there may be only one parent in the home to care for the child. The single parent may be either the father or mother, but is more often the latter. Being the only parent can pose many problems if there is no supportive network of family and friends to assist, especially if the parent must go out to work. Some women decide not to marry but to become mothers and bring up their children independently, making arrangements for the care of the children.

Many Afro-Caribbean children have grown up with the mother the only parent in the home, a tradition from the days of slavery. There has always been a high rate of unemployment in the Caribbean countries and men have had to migrate in search of work. They went from rural to urban areas, from island to island, to the United States, Canada, Cuba, Panama and some South American countries, to the Netherlands Antilles, and recently to Britain. Fathers being absent, the relationship between mothers and children tended to become very close. Edith Clarke, anthropologist, has given the close bond between mother and son as one of the reasons why some young Jamaican men refuse to marry or form close relationships with women before the death of their mothers. The same may be said of men in other countries also. Many of them hold the view that their mothers should be properly repaid for all the sacrifices made for them when they were children.

Unplanned families

An adolescent girl may become a mother without planning or preparing for a family. She may be able to remain within the extended family, but on the other hand she may be asked to leave the home because of her parents' anger, shame and disappointment, especially if the pregnancy occurred whilst still at school. The young man named as being responsible for the pregnancy may refuse to accept paternity, or if he does he may be unemployed, young and inexperienced. His mother may take the child into the family home, but many young mothers prefer to keep their babies and may experience many problems if they live alone.

It is not the happiest start in life for mother or baby so it is best to avoid this situation. The Family Planning Centre is always on hand to give caring advice on sex and contraception.

CHILD ABUSE

Most families are able to cope with the everyday problems and the anxieties usually present when caring for helpless infants, but there are times when some parents are unable to cope with the stresses and strains, and in their frustration become violent and inflict injury on the child.

In recent times, in many countries of the world, child abuse seems to have increased considerably. Voluntary organisations for the prevention of cruelty to children, some of which have been in existence for many years, attempt to give parents support and help in dealing with their problems. The sorrow and guilt which follows the death of an abused child is tremendous, not only for the parents, but also for the relatives, neighbours, health visitors, doctors and social workers involved.

It is important to remember that children are not able to choose their parents. It is up to the parents, whatever the type of family unit, to make them glad that they were born into their particular family. A stable and happy family teaches the importance of sharing and co-operating with others, and provides a firm basis when the children eventually go out into the world.

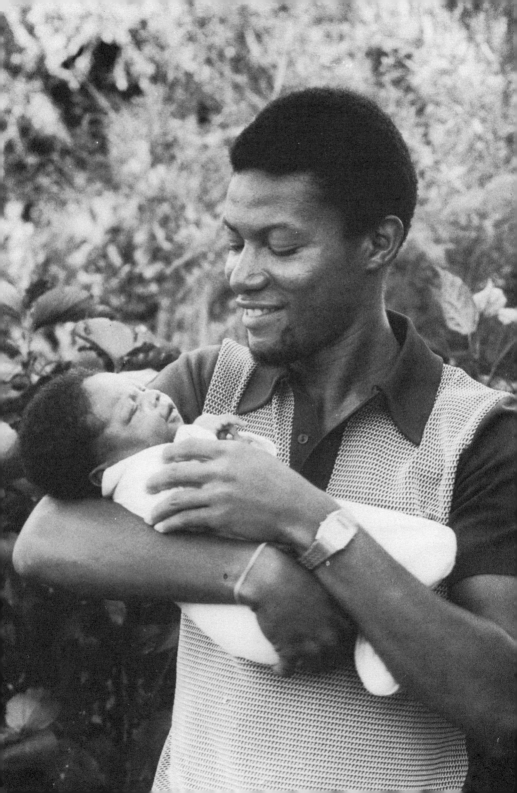

2 Becoming a parent

For most people, starting a family is an important milestone in their lives. The couple experience both joy and anxiety and, if they both accept the responsibility that goes with parenthood, they are able to share those feelings with each other.

FAMILY PLANNING AND HEALTH CLINICS

Family planning plays an important part in the preparation for parenthood because it deals with all the aspects of family life, not only with ways of controlling birth. The aim is to help couples to lead a fuller and less pressured life. If each child in the family is a wanted child, parents are more able to give the attention and care necessary for the children's proper growth and development.

Staff in family planning clinics usually provide information to young men and women about various contraceptive methods, and also deal with other topics such as sexually transmitted diseases, showing how these may be prevented or, if contracted, how they may be treated. Tests are also carried out on women for the detection of breast cancer or cancer of the cervix. All personal details given to the staff at these clinics are treated confidentially.

Years ago, many women died when giving birth, and many babies died before birth. More recently, with increased medical knowledge and improved health facilities, the risk of mothers and babies dying has been greatly reduced, though there are still some countries where, because of poverty or ignorance of proper hygiene or the lack of a balanced diet, pregnant mothers are still very much at risk. In those countries where a system of public health care has been developed (and that includes most Caribbean countries), people are encouraged to make use of the health clinics where great care is taken of pregnant mothers, babies and toddlers.

Being a parent for the first time is a unique experience which most people treasure, but being a good parent is not easy. It is a very demanding job of work and demands a great deal of thought and commitment.

THE ROLE OF MOTHER

The mother is the parent who experiences the greatest changes, physically, emotionally and socially. She may be anxious and worried during the early days of pregnancy, but usually with the birth of a normal healthy baby she becomes more settled.

It is traditional for her to care for the child in its early years. One important reason for this is that she is provided by nature with the means of feeding the baby with milk from her breasts.

During the first few years mother and baby become very close to each other because of the baby's complete dependence on her for food and comfort, and because most mothers accept that they are needed and important to their children. If any other person, such as grandmother, older sister or nursemaid, provides food, care and comfort during this early stage, then the child develops a close relationship with that individual instead of or as well as with the mother.

The mother is usually the child's first teacher. In talking to and playing with her child, she helps his use of language to develop. By the tone of her voice and her facial expression, the baby learns at an early age what pleases and displeases. At the toddler stage mother keeps a close watch while the home and surroundings are explored, and a great deal of imitation takes place. All of this is preparation for formal education at a later date.

The child who is shown love and affection learns to give these in return and develops emotionally. The mother who is firm but kind in her correction, and sets reasonable limits of behaviour, helps in the development of self-discipline. When promises are made and kept, the child learns to trust and the foundation is laid for the development of a trustworthy person.

Caring for a child is a full-time and exacting job during the early years of the child's life. Those who devote the time and energy necessary to do it well are usually rewarded by seeing the children grow up into well-balanced individuals.

BECOMING A PARENT

THE ROLE OF FATHER

The father is important both to the child and to the mother. The emotional support he gives to her helps her to feel at ease within herself and so enables her to care for the child in a relaxed and effective manner. Helping to provide the material needs of the

Before baby is born, father cares ...

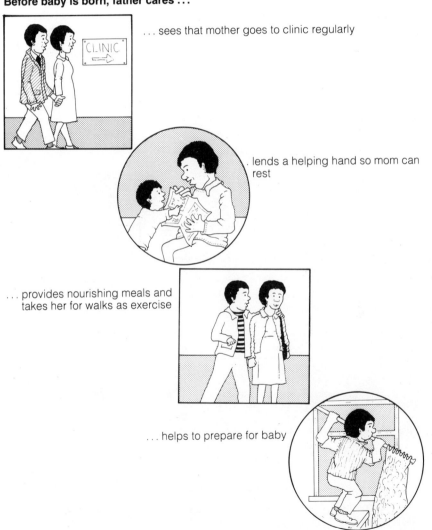

... sees that mother goes to clinic regularly

... lends a helping hand so mom can rest

... provides nourishing meals and takes her for walks as exercise

... helps to prepare for baby

THE FAMILY

family is also important, so that both mother and child may be properly housed, clothed and fed.

Immediately after the birth of the baby father may feel left out, as friends and relatives give most of their attention to mother and baby, but he too can become involved in caring for the child. All of the comforting tasks which are performed by the mother can also be done by the father. He may bottle feed the child when it is weaned from the breast or feed the baby with a mug and spoon when solids are taken. He may also bath and change the child and take him out for walks. In this way, the beginning of a relationship is formed. Indeed, in some families where the mother works it could be the father who is responsible for the early upbringing of the baby.

Father plays a big part when baby arrives ...

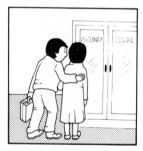

... calls midwife, or takes mother to maternity centre

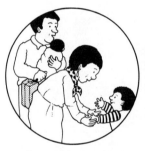

... takes mother and baby home

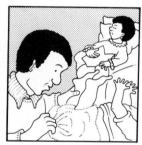

... lends a helping hand so mother can rest

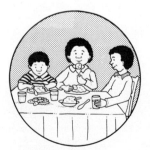

... sees mother gets nourishing meals

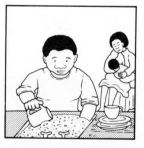

... assists in the home

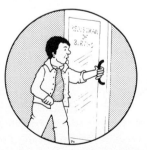

... registers baby's birth

BECOMING A PARENT

For infant and mother care, father ...

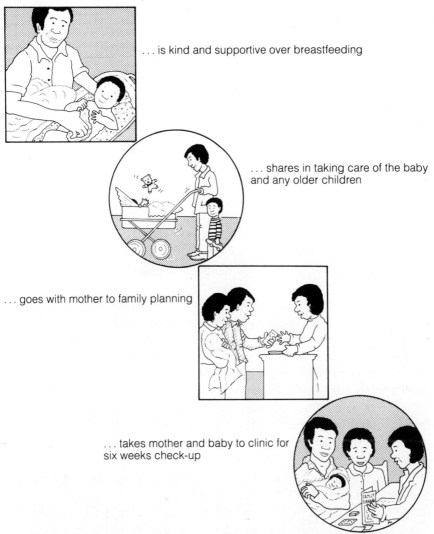

... is kind and supportive over breastfeeding

... shares in taking care of the baby and any older children

... goes with mother to family planning

... takes mother and baby to clinic for six weeks check-up

    The father's interest in the child helps to build a feeling of well-being in the family. The example of mother and father sharing in the life of the home helps to provide some reference for the future when the child becomes an adult and starts his own family.

    In many societies the father in the family tends to leave the responsibility of bringing up the children entirely to the mother, saying that looking after children is 'women's business'. But fathering is similar to mothering. Both terms mean loving, caring, teaching the child, setting examples. They mean sharing pleasures and pain with the child, taking an interest in every aspect of its growth and development, and building a warm and affectionate relationship which will last as long as life itself.

STEP-PARENTS

A mother or father who is not the natural parent of the child in the family is called a **step-parent**. Depending on the age of the child or children, the step-parent may or may not be welcomed into the family easily.

The loss of a parent affects the child in some way. A baby may miss the face or sound of the parent's voice which was just becoming familiar; the toddler who may not fully understand death may still hope for the parent's return; an older child may feel guilty and in some way responsible if his father or mother had left through a divorce.

A fairy-tale 'Cinderella' known to many children in the western world which paints a picture of the bad stepmother, has caused negative attitudes towards stepmothers. But many stepmothers have wonderful relationships with their stepchildren.

As with all human relationships, there is need for mutual trust and this only develops gradually if the step-parent is prepared to make changes slowly and allow the children to keep some of their favourite belongings about the house, if they wish, to remind them of their absent parent. Baby and stepmother will respond well to each other if the one gives the care that the other needs. If the stepfather has been a bachelor for most of his adult life and is unable to tolerate a young child and its demands, or is resentful of another man's child, there may be problems, especially if the family is a nuclear one and there are no relatives available to share the care of the child. In extreme cases, the mother may be forced to make other arrangements for the child.

There are times when older children find difficulty in knowing how to address the step-parent, not wanting to use the term 'mum' or 'dad' by which they had called their own parents. Where there is reluctance to accept the step-parent, the adolescent may insist on being formal and address him or her as 'Mr' or 'Mrs', to the embarrassment of the natural parent. The atmosphere in the home may become so strained that finally the adolescent may leave the family.

As children grow older, there may be jealousy between the surviving parent and the child of the same sex who sees him or herself as a rival for the step-parent's attention. There are some instances where male step-parents encourage relationships between themselves and stepdaughters and cause great hurt and emotional disturbance in the girls and their mothers who may be too embarrassed to talk about the problem. The family situation can be very unpleasant and unhappy.

Some step-parents find the task of keeping a family together extremely difficult as resentful and angry feelings, which are also present in natural families at times, seem to increase, especially if there are children of both partners. The surviving partner may fantasise about the absent one's virtues. He or she and the children may make comparisons about the cooking or the caring, or the amount of money that was available, saying: 'Everything somehow used to be better.' Instead of bottling up hurt feelings the individuals should talk these over with a trusted friend or with an experienced social worker.

However, if the step-parents are emotionally mature they will treat the children as if they were the natural parents, or simply good friends, and the family will be happy and stable.

ADOPTIVE PARENTS

A permanent arrangement of providing other parents is by means of adoption. The agencies that arrange adoptions may pay great attention to their selection of **adoptive parents**, and try to ensure that the applicants are physically and mentally well, of good character and without a criminal record, and that they love children and are able to care for them in every possible way. The adoptive parents' ability to show warmth and affection for a child is much more important than their financial standing.

Adoption is a very serious undertaking and in order to help both parents and child relate to each other, the child is placed for a trial period of several months (the length of time may vary from country to country) before the arrangement is made legal. During this time, regular visits are made by the adoption worker who observes how the child settles in the family, and discusses any problems which the new parents may be experiencing. This trial period can be a very anxious time because the natural parent(s) may have second thoughts on the matter and refuse to give consent. Obviously, this anxiety will not arise if the child is an orphan.

As soon as the adoption worker is confident that the adoptive parents and child are happy with each other, and the necessary consent from the natural parent(s) is obtained, an Adoption Order is made in a court of law and the child is registered with the surname of its adoptive parents. When this is done the natural parents no longer have any legal rights over the child.

In the early days of formal adoption, it was the practice to keep the fact of adoption a well-guarded secret from the children. This caused a lot of problems, especially if they were told by others that the parents whom they called mother and father were not their real parents. Nowadays in most countries this has changed and children are told as soon as they are capable of understanding why they were adopted. After all, one of the meanings of the word 'adopt' is 'choose' and, when children realise that their adoptive parents have chosen them, they feel wanted.

Many adopted children, when grown-up, are curious to find their natural parents and often seek them out. The search may go on for a very long time and great disappointment may be experienced if the parents are not found, or if, when found, they do not fit their expectations. But sometimes, the reunion of parent and child can be a delight to them both, with the adoptive parent sharing in their joy.

FOSTER PARENTS

There are times when parents are unable to care for their children, and relatives, friends or neighbours, or carefully selected strangers act as substitute parents. They are commonly known as **foster parents**. Fostering is a common practice throughout the Caribbean where relatives or friends with or without their own children readily take a child into their family. The natural parents are free to visit and may contribute financially if they are able to do so. In many instances the arrangements are satisfactory and the foster parents and child become attached to each other. One disadvantage of such an informal arrangement is that children may be moved from home to home depending on the whims of one or both parents, and consequently suffer from a lack of security and experience difficulty in forming close and lasting relationships with adults.

In some Caribbean countries, governments make more formal arrangements, and, through their Child Care or Social Service Departments, accept responsibility for the care of the children who they place with selected foster parents. The natural parents give their consent, and in most instances are encouraged to visit. Visits may not be allowed if there has been a poor relationship between parents and children. All financial arrangements are taken care of officially, but money can never compensate for the loving care and affection which are given to the children.

There may be times when the situation of the natural parents improves and they wish to have their children rejoin their family group. This very often poses problems if the children have become attached to the foster parents and they to the children. Both sets of parents need to be helped to understand this and give the children time to make the break. Short visits home to natural parents may be arranged at first and gradually the time increased. After returning home the child may be allowed to visit the foster parents.

CHILDREN'S HOMES

There are times when adoptive or foster parents are not available, or parents think they may only need temporary help in looking after the children. In some such cases children are placed in a children's home. If the home caters for a small number of children and resembles as closely as possible an ordinary home with a couple as house-mother and house-father, family life can be experienced. Unfortunately, this ideal set-up is not often possible. Homes cater for large numbers of children, and house-parents work in shifts. The children are not able to form a special, close relationship with any adult, and this can set an unhappy pattern for all future relationships. That is why there is a growing practice in homes to encourage people in the community to become 'uncles' and 'aunts' to the children, who benefit from the individual attention.

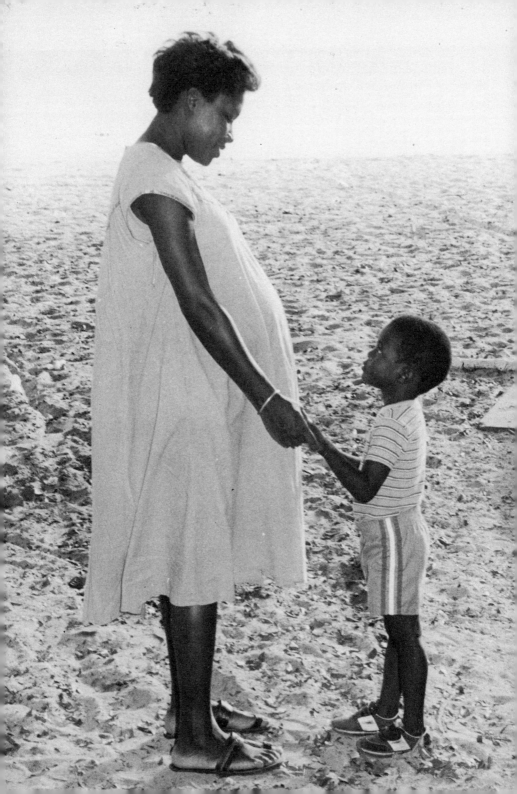

PART TWO: HOW HUMAN LIFE BEGINS

3 Where do babies come from?

It is estimated that two babies are born every second somewhere in the world. That means 120 human beings every minute. Human life begins with the union of the mother's egg with the sperm cell of the father. It is difficult to believe that human life starts from such small beginnings!

The human body is wonderfully made. It grows in stages, each stage being a preparation for the next. It contains organs specially designed to perform specific functions. Slowly and gradually changes take place within the body through childhood and adolescence until it matures into adulthood.

The stage of growth when boys and girls develop into being physically capable of becoming parents is known as **puberty**. Puberty usually begins around age 12 in girls and 14 in boys, but may be earlier or later as each individual develops at his or her own rate. This does not mean, however, that the adolescent or teenager is sufficiently mature emotionally to start a family. Adolescence is a time of change, not only in body but in mind, when boys and girls strive to be independent. Sometimes everything seems to go well, whilst at other times everything goes wrong and feelings are low and changeable. Teenagers are often difficult to live with in the family. But if the family is one where parents and children have always communicated with each other, good, bad and confused feelings may be shared and discussed. Sometimes the adolescent may choose to confide in another relative or family friend or in a trusted adult outside the family.

Being an adolescent is not always easy, but it is an interesting time in the life of an individual, and the young man or woman knows that it is a step towards becoming an adult.

HORMONAL CHANGES IN THE ADOLESCENT

Men and women each have two sex glands. In women they are called **ovaries**, and in men, **testicles**. These glands contain thousands of tiny cells. They secrete chemical substances called hormones which enter the bloodstream and are circulated through the body.

During puberty the female sex glands release two different hormones:

1. **Oestrogen**: this causes the female sex organs to develop; the breasts enlarge, and hair grows in the armpits and over the pubic bone.
2. **Progesterone**: this mainly affects the **uterus** or womb, and prepares it for holding a baby.

The male sex glands produce the hormone called **testosterone**. Circulating through the bloodstream and therefore to all parts of the body, it causes the boy's appearance to change. The sex organs develop, hair may grow on his face and under his arms and over his pubic bone and, in some boys, on the chest. The shoulders broaden and generally he becomes more muscular, and his voice becomes deeper.

THE FEMALE REPRODUCTIVE ORGANS

The uterus: a woman has the important function of carrying the baby so her body contains the organ for this purpose, the **uterus**. The uterus lies inside the body between the bowel and the bladder. It is hollow and pear-shaped and is about seven-and-a-half centimetres long. The narrow neck is called the **cervix**. The cervix leads into the **vagina** which is the passage out of the body. The walls of the uterus are made of thick muscles which are able to expand as the baby grows inside it.

The ovaries: there are two ovaries, one on either side of the uterus, and each contains thousands of tiny female cells called **ova** or eggs. Only a few hundred of these will mature during a woman's lifetime.

The Fallopian tubes: the Fallopian tubes or **oviducts** lead out from each of the upper corners of the uterus and look like two

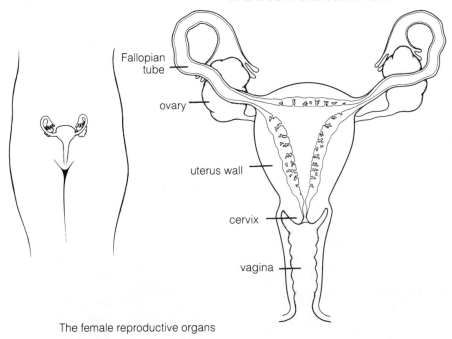

The female reproductive organs

arms with fingers at both ends. It is through these tubes that the ova pass from the ovaries to the uterus.

MENSTRUATION

This is a physical change which is a necessary part of growing up, and is the term for the monthly discharge of blood from the uterus through the vagina. About once a month the pituitary gland, which is situated at the base of the brain, secretes a hormone which causes an ovum to ripen. This ripened egg pushes its way out of the ovary; this is called **ovulation**. Whilst the egg is travelling from the ovary, the lining of the uterus thickens, preparing a special layer of blood vessels and tissues to nourish the egg. If sexual intercourse takes place at this time and the egg is fertilised by the male cell it will attach itself to the lining and develop into a baby. If not fertilised, it passes out of the body. Since the lining of the uterus is not required it stops growing and loosens. The blood vessels come away from the walls of the uterus and bleed. The blood flows through the vagina out of the body. This is called the

HOW HUMAN LIFE BEGINS

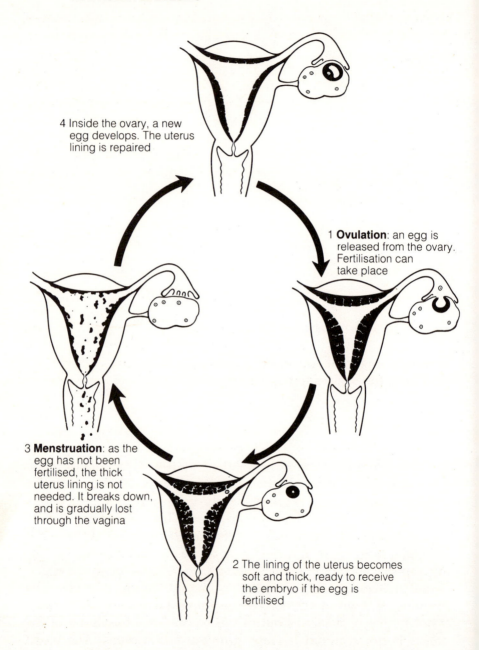

The menstrual cycle

menstrual flow or monthly period, and may last from three to seven days. It usually occurs every 28 days but the cycle may vary in some people from 21 to 35 days. The days are counted from the beginning of one period to the start of the next.

The age at which menstruation starts also varies. Usually it begins between the ages of 11 and 14, but it can begin earlier or later. Periods are not always regular in the first year, but as time goes by a regular pattern generally emerges. Sometimes physical illness, or emotional anxieties over a special event like sitting an examination, may cause the periods to be irregular. However, if the irregularity persists over any length of time, it should be discussed with a doctor.

Sometimes, periods are accompanied by feelings of depression, tiredness or tension. This is known as **pre-menstrual tension**, and it varies considerably from girl to girl: some experience nothing at all; others may have to lie down for a day or stop their normal activities for a short while.

Provided there are no abnormalities or removal of any of the reproductive organs because of disease, menstruation continues (except during pregnancy) until a woman reaches her late 40s or early 50s, sometimes earlier, sometimes later. Then the periods gradually stop. This is known as the **menopause** or the **change** and may cause tension or depression in some women.

Myths

There are many myths connected with menstruation, caused no doubt by a misunderstanding of what really happens. Some people regarded it as an illness, others that the woman was unclean and therefore she should not mix with others or do the cooking until the end of the period. Still others thought it was harmful to bath during those days. Fortunately in most of our societies, with improved knowledge, young people know that these myths are not true.

Personal hygiene during menstruation

Personal hygiene is very important during this time, and a daily bath with the water at a comfortable warm temperature is very soothing. Clothes we kept clean by wearing a sanitary napkin (or tampon, which is worn internally) to soak up the flow. Being disposable, they can be changed easily and frequently. In some rural areas people still use cloth sanitary napkins; if these are washed in cold water immediately after use no ugly stains remain. There is no reason why the average healthy young woman should not enjoy any form of sport or physical activity during menstruation.

Dysmenorrhea

Dysmenorrhea (pronounced dis-men-o-ria) is the medical term used for pain during menstruation. The majority of girls and women experience very little pain or none at all. There may be a slight feeling of heaviness or cramps during the first day of the period, and a feeling of listlessness or irritability. Normally this disappears quite early on in the period, but if constant and severe pains continue, the doctor should be consulted. There may be a physical cause, or the pains may be caused by tension and fear especially if the girl does not know what is happening to her. Others may know what is happening, but may be afraid of growing up. If the tension is through fear, it would be wise for the girl to try to confide in someone she trusts. Menstruation is a normal stage in the life of a woman and the majority experience little stress and continue their activities normally during it.

THE MALE REPRODUCTIVE ORGANS

The male reproductive organs are designed to do three things:

- manufacture sperms in the testicles
- deposit sperms as close to the cervix as possible
- manufacture the male sex hormone, testosterone

They are made up of the following parts:
The penis: This is the organ through which the male deposits sperms at the top of the vagina. It consists mainly of erectile tissue which under the influence of sexual excitement becomes filled and engorged with blood so the organ becomes rigid and can ejaculate sperms out through the male's urethra and into the female vagina during copulation.

The testicles: These are suspended beneath the penis in the scrotum. They are oval in shape. They produce sperms and the male hormone testosterone.

The scrotum: This is a bag of loose skin containing the testicles which is suspended behind the penis.

The prostate and seminal vesicles: The **prostate** is a gland situated at the base of the penis. The **seminal vesicles** are attached to the prostate, one on each side. The prostate and seminal vesicles manufacture the seminal fluid in which sperms can survive indefinitely.

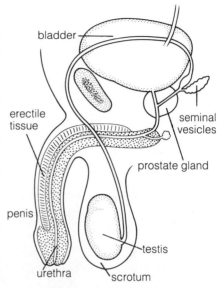

The male reproductive organs

Seminal emission

Sometimes in adolescence, during sleep, as a result of a sexually exciting dream, ejaculation takes place when the seminal fluid suddenly passes out from the body through the erect penis. This is described as a **'wet dream'**. Boys may be alarmed when this happens for the first time and need to be prepared for it – and reassured that it is a normal occurrence in growing up.

THE SEXUAL ACT

When the erect male penis enters the female vagina and ejaculates the seminal fluid containing sperms, then **sexual intercourse** is said to have taken place. Sometimes, when this happens for the first time for a girl or woman, slight bleeding occurs and the girl may experience mild pain as the skin lying across the vaginal entrance, the **hymen,** is stretched or torn. If it is torn, the girl may experience slight discomfort during intercourse until it heals. Sometimes the hymen can be stretched and broken away before sexual intercourse has ever taken place – in the normal process of growing up.

CONCEPTION

The life of a new human being begins when a male sex cell enters the female cell and joins with it to form one cell. This is called **fertilisation**. When sexual intercourse occurs, millions of sperms in seminal fluid pass from the testicles out through the urethra in the penis and enter the vagina of the woman. The tiny cells swim swiftly through the cervix into the uterus and on through the Fallopian tubes. If there is an ovum in the tube, one of the sperm cells can enter it.

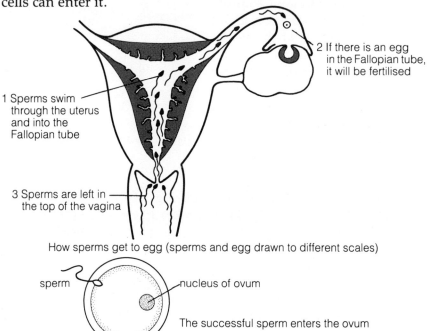

1 Sperms swim through the uterus and into the Fallopian tube

2 If there is an egg in the Fallopian tube, it will be fertilised

3 Sperms are left in the top of the vagina

How sperms get to egg (sperms and egg drawn to different scales)

sperm   nucleus of ovum

The successful sperm enters the ovum

SEXUALLY TRANSMITTED DISEASES (VENEREAL DISEASE)

Young people should think very carefully before deciding to enter a sexual union and need to be fully aware of the physical consequences. One consequence may be the girl's pregnancy, for which the couple may not be ready, and another could be the contracting of a sexually transmitted disease (if one or the other has had intercourse with other partners).

These diseases are widespread and are caused by germs

which spread only through intimate physical contact, mainly sexual, with an infected person. They are not contracted by sitting on lavatory seats as some people think.

The danger of sexually transmitted diseases is that they may be present without the boy or girl knowing until some complication of the disease arises. Two of the most prevalent diseases are **syphilis** and **gonorrhea** but all of these diseases are seriously harmful to the body. Some can be transmitted by the mother to the unborn child, so it is extremely important to seek help from family planning clinics – where check-ups are completely confidential – if there is the slightest possibility of having contracted the disease.

Even more worrying is the growing incidence of Aids (Acquired Immune Deficiency Syndrome). At present there is no known cure for this fatal disease. It can also be transmitted from the mother to the unborn child.

PLEASE ... see a doctor if you suspect you have AIDS.

From a leaflet prepared by the Bureau of Health Education, Kingston, Jamaica

---

WHAT'S AIDS?

Well, it's a disease by which the body loses its ability to protect itself from everyday germs. Germs that wouldn't ordinarily cause death, will do so in the case of an AIDS victim.

HOW'S AIDS SPREAD?

Now that's the cruncher!... doctors believe AIDS is spread mainly through sexual contact. After all, over 75% of all AIDS victims are homosexual or bisexual men.

Avoid having sex with prostitutes

Avoid quickly formed sexual relationships ... especially with folks whose sexual preferences and hygiene we know little or nothing about

Avoid anal sex (using the rectum for sex)

Use a condom

Avoid swallowing semen, urine and faeces

There is proof too, that the disease may be caught through

needles shared with infected drug addicts

transfusion of blood or blood components from AIDS victims ... and

PLEASE...those of us who are homosexual or bisexual (having sex with both male and female) should give up... GIVING BLOOD.

BUT THAT'S NOT ALL...infected moms can pass AIDS to their babies.

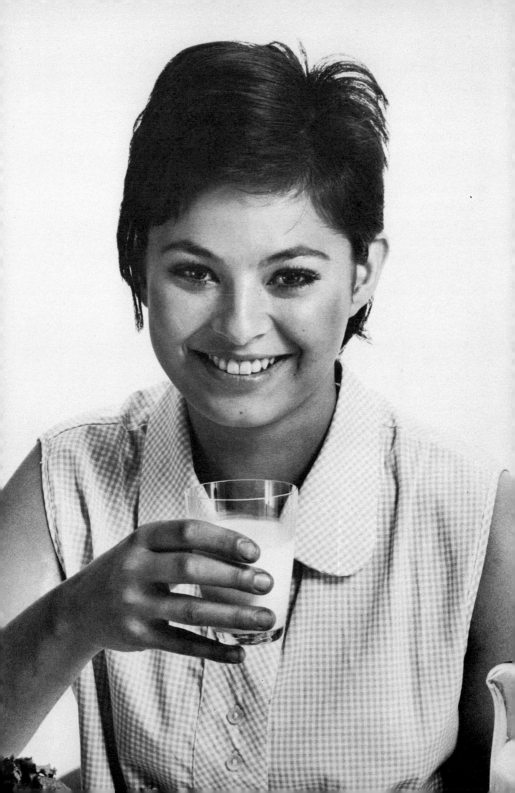

4 Pre-natal development

During the first few hours after fertilisation of the ovum by the sperm, the **nucleus** (the result of the fusion of the male and female **nuclei**) enlarges and moves towards the centre of the ovum. Soon the fused nucleus divides into two equal parts, and then further subdivides to form a cluster of cells called the **embryo**.

THE PROGRESS OF THE FERTILISED OVUM

About seven days after fertilisation, the embryo enters the cavity of the uterus and sinks into the soft lining. Now the embryo begins to differentiate into its various parts and after eight weeks is called a **foetus**. The baby is fully formed by the end of the twelfth week of pregnancy, and from then on it only grows and matures, although none of the organs is sufficiently developed to function independently.

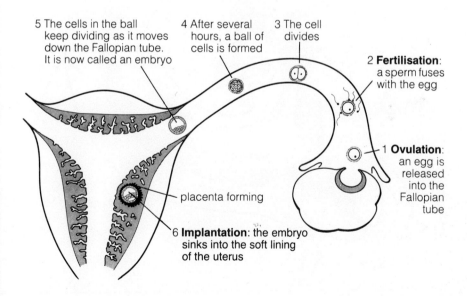

Stages leading to implantation

THE PLACENTA

At the point where the fertilised ovum becomes attached to the uterus wall, a very important organ, the **placenta**, is formed. The placenta is a circular flesh-like substance covered by a thin transparent membrane through which the mother's blood nourishes the foetus. Inside this membrane is a fluid called the **amniotic fluid** which surrounds the baby as it grows and is important for the following reasons:

- It allows the baby to move about inside the uterus
- It protects the baby from the bumps caused by the everyday activity of the mother

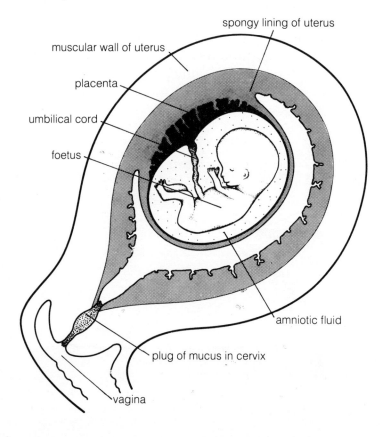

Side view of developing embryo foetus inside uterus

THE UMBILICAL CORD

The baby is attached to the placenta by a narrow cord known as the **umbilical cord**, commonly called the 'navel string'. It contains two arteries and a vein through which nutrients and oxygen from the mother's blood and the waste products of the baby are exchanged. The mother's blood and the baby's blood are kept separate – only the nutrients and oxygen from the mother and the waste products from the baby are exchanged. After the birth of the baby, the cord is tied and cut. (When the spot heals and dries a few weeks later, this becomes the navel.) The placenta detaches itself from the uterus wall and follows the path of the baby out of the vagina – this is known as the **afterbirth**. This is then disposed of.

DEVELOPMENT OF THE FOETUS

When a woman conceives, she and her partner will naturally be interested in how the baby is developing. This chart shows the average development rate of the foetus in the womb.

4 weeks	Beginning of the formation of the internal organs: the heart, brain, liver, lungs.
5 weeks	The backbone is forming, the head grows rapidly, the limb buds show the beginnings of arms and legs.
6 weeks	The arms and legs are recognisable, with webbed fingers and toes.
7 weeks	Ears and eyelids begin to grow. The internal organs are moving into place.
3 months	The fingers and toes are well-formed.
4 months	The nails begin to show on the well-formed fingers and toes. The milk teeth are forming in the gums. A little hair begins to show on the scalp.
5 months	The first faint heartbeat may be heard through the doctor's stethoscope.

HOW HUMAN LIFE BEGINS

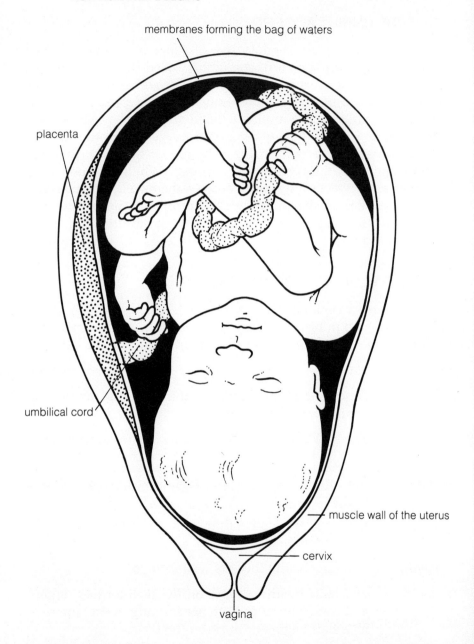

Full-term baby in birth position

PRE-NATAL DEVELOPMENT

6 months   The baby's movements may be felt. She changes position. Sometimes the head is up, sometimes down. Sometimes she is quiet, suggesting that she may be asleep.

7 months   A soft creamy substance called **vernix** begins to cover the body. Sometimes a baby is born at this stage. Although her arrival is unexpected, there is a good chance of survival.

8–9 months   The bones of the skull become harder, hair begins to grow longer. The cartilage of the nose and ears develops. The nails grow beyond the tips of the fingers and toes.

Normally the head is down towards the cervix. The baby is ready for birth. When born at this time the baby is described as a **full-term baby**.

INHERITED FACTORS

The sex of the child

Once the pregnancy is confirmed, many expectant parents wonder about the sex of the child. Some may have a preference for one or other of the sexes and, among some cultures, it is very important that the firstborn is a boy. However, the sex of the child is fixed at conception, and although a great deal of research has gone into ways of producing a male or female child to order, no real practical progress has been made.

All human cells contain 46 **chromosomes** which determine the inherited characteristics of the individual. 22 pairs of chromosomes in the cells are identical, but the 23rd pair – the sex chromosomes – are different in the male and female. Females have two X chromosomes while males have one X and one Y chromosome. When the sperm fertilises the ovum, the father supplies 23 chromosomes and the mother the other 23. Each ovum contains one X chromosome, while half the male sperms contain an X and the other half a Y chromosome. If the ovum containing the X is fertilised by a sperm containing an X chromosome, the new cell will have two X chromosomes and will be a girl. If, however, the ovum is fertilised by a sperm containing the Y chromosome, the new cell will have an X and a Y chromosome and the baby will be a boy.

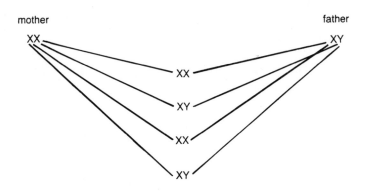

How the sex of the child is determined – as shown in the diagram it is a 50/50 chance whether the baby will be a boy or a girl

Family traits

What will the baby be like? Will she be tall or short? Will she have blue or brown eyes? Will she have light or dark skin? Every chromosome contains a set of **genes** which determine the characteristics of the baby and future individual. While some characteristics, such as body build and personality, will be affected by external factors, certain characteristics, such as colour of eyes, curly hair etc., cannot be changed. Where, for example, both parents have curly hair, the children are practically certain to have curly hair. The baby inherits 50 per cent from the father and 50 per cent from the mother so, although she may resemble the parents in many respects, she has a unique combination of genes which make her into a unique individual.

Since many families in Caribbean countries have ancestors of several races, it is possible for a child to look different from her parents in skin colour since she may have inherited characteristics from a grandparent through her parents.

INHERITED DISEASES: SICKLE CELL ANAEMIA

Some diseases can be passed down from one generation to another. One such condition, that is fairly common in Caribbean countries is **sickle cell disease**. This is so-called because the normally rounded red blood cells become crescent or sickle-shaped when they give up their oxygen.

It usually causes severe anaemia from about the age of six months. Because of the sickle shape of the red cells they tend to block the small blood vessels, causing pain which can be very severe and sometimes leads to permanent damage and even death. People with sickle cell anaemia are also more prone to coughs, colds, sore throats and other serious infections.

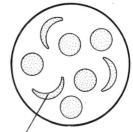

The crescent-shaped sickle cell

How sickle cell anaemia is inherited

Sickle cell occurs as a result of a deformity of a substance called **haemoglobin**, a constituent of the red blood cells. The most common type of haemoglobin is Haemoglobin A (HbA), and most people inherit this from both parents. Occasionally something goes wrong and sperms and eggs may develop the sickle cell type of haemoglobin (HbS). These sperms and eggs can then pass on the disease to future offspring. The drawing shows how this disease is inherited. Some people can pass the disease on to their offspring without suffering from it themselves. These people are called carriers.

If one parent has normal HbA and the other HbS (is a carrier), none of the children will suffer from sickle cell anaemia, but there is a chance that one out of every two children will be a carrier.

If, however, both parents are carriers, the chances are that one out of every four children will have sickle cell anaemia, one out of every two will be a carrier, and one will be normal.

HOW HUMAN LIFE BEGINS

How sickle cell anaemia is inherited

A This is what happens if a carrier marries a normal person

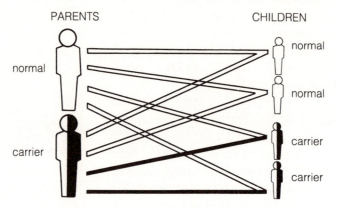

None of these children suffer from sickle cell anaemia but two are carriers

B This is what happens if a carrier marries another carrier

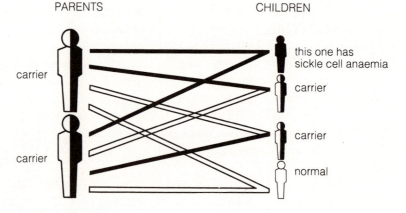

MULTIPLE BIRTHS

A few mothers have three, four or more babies at a time, especially with the increasing use of fertility drugs. This never fails to be of great interest to many people, and especially to the media. Twins are more common, but having twins usually runs in families.

There are two kinds of twins, **fraternal** and **identical**. Fraternal twins are different babies from the time of conception. They come from two separate ova, each one being separately fertilised. Each baby has its own placenta. These babies are just as different as other brothers and sisters.

Identical twins begin as a fertilised single ovum, but when the new single cell begins to divide, the two halves separate. Each of the new cells thus formed has all the powers of life and growth. The two babies are usually attached to the same placenta, but in some cases each may have its own. However, they have separate umbilical cords and separate bags of water. The babies are always of the same sex and so much alike that sometimes even the parents have difficulty in telling them apart, and usually distinguish them in some way. When twins are growing up, they sometimes use this resemblance to their own advantage in playing tricks on their friends, teachers and parents. However, it is important to treat each child as an individual.

INFERTILITY

There are times when a healthy couple who love children and would like to have them are unable to do so. The causes may be physical or emotional and may be found in the man, or the woman, or both. A thorough examination of both partners and laboratory tests often determine if there is a physical cause which can be treated. There are times when treatment with fertility drugs may produce results far above the doctor's or the couple's expectations, and multiple births of as many as six babies (sextuplets) can result. If the infertility is due to emotional problems, counselling is tried in order to discover the cause. Often, if the couple decide to adopt a baby, the wife then becomes pregnant. This is probably because the wife becomes more relaxed and at ease within herself and is then emotionally ready for pregnancy.

It was mistakenly believed that infertility was caused by the female partner's inability to conceive. But this is not true: infertility is a problem in men as well. Both partners should consult the doctor.

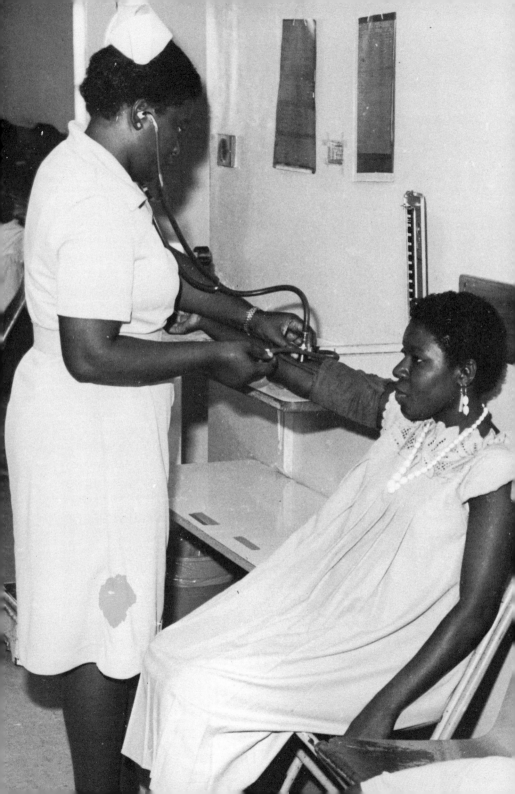

5 Pregnancy

Knowing how the reproductive organs function and being able to answer the question 'Where do babies come from?' does not mean that an individual is ready to become a parent. Young men and women, through keeping themselves interested in physical, intellectual and creative activities, by doing some sort of work (whether paid or voluntary) are usually able to control their sexual instincts. This is known as **sublimation**. It is to their advantage to delay entering 'the family way' until they are emotionally mature, that is, until they are able to devote time and attention, and to give love and affection to someone other than themselves. It is also essential that they can financially support the child.

UNDERSTANDING THE CHANGES

If two people who have a close relationship with each other based on love, understanding and mutual trust, decide to start a family, they need to prepare themselves for change. Some of the changes are:

1. **The physical change of the woman**: she may be very pleased and accept the changes in her body, or may regret the loss of her figure. The man may also be reluctant to take her out socially, until her figure returns to normal after the birth of the baby. This attitude can lead to problems in the relationship.

2. **Change of lifestyle**: pregnancy is not an illness, but at times there may be some indisposition which prevents the pregnant woman from working or taking part in the couple's social or domestic activities.

3. **Emotional changes**: anxiety about the added responsibilities may cause changes of mood in both partners, making them irritable with each other. Fortunately, there is help available at antenatal clinics, and it is important that it is accepted from the earliest stage.

THE FIRST SIGNS OF PREGNANCY

The woman's body undergoes substantial changes. The monthly periods usually stop, the breasts become enlarged and tender when touched. As the uterus grows, the bladder, with the pressure upon it, becomes more active and there is the need to empty it more regularly. Some women have increased secretion of saliva and tend to spit frequently. The figure becomes more rounded and some relatives or friends refer to a young woman's pregnancy by saying 'she is fat'.

A woman may also experience **morning sickness**. The precise cause is not known but some women may experience nausea (the feeling that usually precedes vomiting). These bad feelings may occur at any time of the day, although they seem to be more frequent during the morning, hence the name morning sickness. A doctor is consulted if the nausea is severe or lasts too long after the first three months of pregnancy, when it can normally be expected to stop.

In order to be quite sure of pregnancy, the doctor is consulted and, besides a physical examination, samples of urine are taken for laboratory tests.

ANTENATAL CARE: STATE AND MEDICAL

Years ago, lack of medical knowledge and adequate antenatal care meant that other things went wrong during pregnancy. Nowadays, women are advised to go for regular monthly checks from the beginning of the pregnancy until the time of delivery. At the antenatal clinic the following routine checks take place:

1 **Blood**: blood samples are taken at the beginning of the pregnancy to check for blood type, syphilis, and anaemia. These can then be treated if necessary.

2 **Urine**: a urine specimen is examined to check that the kidneys are functioning properly, and that the woman is not suffering from diabetes.

3 **Blood pressure**: this is routinely checked for if it rises too high above the normal level, it may be a sign of kidney or heart disease, or it may cause problems late on in the pregnancy.

4 **Increase in weight**: too large an increase in weight may cause the blood pressure to rise during the late stages of the pregnancy, or too small an increase might mean that the baby is not growing properly.

5 **Abdominal examination**: this is known as **palpation**. It is usually carried out by the **obstetrician** (a specialist in pregnancy and delivery). The size of the uterus and the position of the baby are assessed. If necessary, it is possible to turn the baby round so that it is in the correct birth position.

6 **Vaginal examination**: this is done on the first visit to the antenatal clinic. Obstetricians can then find out if there is anything wrong so that it can be treated in time. The size of the pelvis is also assessed to ensure the baby has enough room to pass through during delivery.

If the doctor thinks it is necessary to see how the baby is developing in the uterus, this is possible with a special test known as an **ultrasound scan**. It gives an image of the baby inside the mother's uterus.

The doctor and the nurses at the clinics also take an interest in the emotional state of the expectant mother, and answer any questions which may be causing her anxiety. They help in calculating the time of the delivery of the baby. Fathers are also welcomed and are free to ask questions, but many men think that antenatal care concerns only the mothers, and only accompany them if specially asked by the doctor or nurse to do so. On the other hand, those fathers who may be willing to attend antenatal classes may not be able to get time off from work. Perhaps when it is more widely accepted that the child is the responsibility of two people, more employers will be persuaded to give paternity leave to those who request it, in the same way that maternity leave is given.

Practical demonstrations

The health visitors at the clinic encourage the mother to join relaxation classes where the breathing exercises that will be important during delivery of the baby are demonstrated. Practical demonstrations about the care of a young child are given: bathing the baby; fitting diapers; mixing feeds; cleaning and sterilising bottles and other feeding utensils. There are also discussions about breast feeding and its advantages.

The relationship which develops between the health visitor and the pregnant mother through regular attendance at the clinic is invaluable, especially during delivery and in the first few weeks afterwards. This is built on a feeling of trust in someone who knows her and is interested in her welfare.

The pregnant working mother

In many countries the working mother has the right to time off work, with pay, to attend antenatal clinics. Proper arrangements need to be made with the employer so that there is no unpleasant argument about being absent when appointments are due. Maternity leave from work usually starts 11 weeks before the baby is due and mothers may return within 29 weeks of the week in which the baby is born. Some working mothers may choose to stay at home for a longer period or give up work altogether, as long as they are able to manage financially.

Time of arrival of the baby

The time when the baby is due to arrive is calculated by counting 40 weeks or 280 days from the date of the first day of the last menstrual period. For example, if the date was 4 March, then the baby is due on 8 December. Some babies, especially the first, may be late in arriving. As has been stressed, events in the lives of human beings do not happen like clockwork. It can be a very anxious time for mother and father if the baby is late, and the support of doctors and the health visitor is particularly appreciated at this time.

SELF-CARE DURING PREGNANCY

There are many things a woman can do for herself to ensure she is fit and well for the delivery.

Guide to Healthy Eating

✶ Cut down on fat, sugar and salt.

✶ Eat more fibre-rich foods.

✶ Eat plenty of fresh fruit and vegetables.

✶ Go easy on alcohol.

✶ Get plenty of variety in what you eat.

✶ If you follow this guide to healthy eating, you'll be getting all the health-giving protein, vitamins and minerals you need.

Nutrition

Proper nutrition (eating foods in a balanced diet) is important not only for the mother but also for the developing baby. Malnutrition is caused by not eating enough of the right food in proper quantities. This condition retards the physical growth of the baby, and can cause mental retardation. In those countries of the world where there is severe poverty, many children suffer severely from the effects of malnutrition, and even in developed countries there are instances where, through unemployment, parents are unable to provide sufficient or nutritious food. Sometimes, through ignorance of the value of foods, children are fed with too many starchy foods and not given a balanced diet.

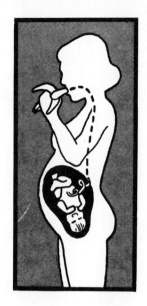

A balanced diet provides the essential nutrients in correct quantities. These are:

- **Protein** for body-building and repairing worn-out tissue
- **Carbohydrates** and **fats** to provide energy and warmth
- **Minerals** to help in the building of bone tissue, red blood cells and body tissue
- **Vitamins** to help promote healthy skin, good eyesight, to help digestion and assist in maintaining the body in a healthy state
- **Roughage** to prevent constipation
- **Adequate fluid** to maintain normal hydration

Overeating

The idea that the expectant mother needs to 'eat for two' is mistaken. She needs only to eat in quantities that satisfy her, and the baby will be sufficiently nourished. Putting on extra weight by eating too many sweets, biscuits and cakes should also be avoided, so as to prevent any undue strain on vital organs such as the heart.

PREGNANCY

Mother's health depends mainly on the food she eats

Eat A Mixture Of Foods At Every Meal

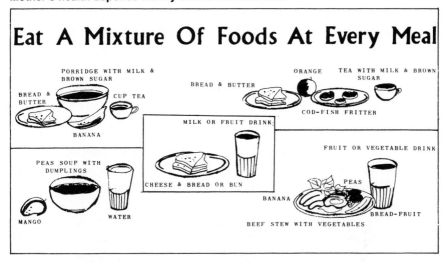

A healthy mother has a better chance of having a healthy baby because the unborn baby is nourished by the food the mother eats
From 'Food for the Expectant Mother', the Bureau of Health Education, Kingston, Jamaica

Cravings

During pregnancy the expectant mother may have a craving and longing for certain foods either sour or sweet, or substances such as charcoal and chalk. Relatives and friends often jokingly warn the mother not to touch any part of her body when expressing the desire, for there is the belief that the baby will bear a birth mark resembling the desired item on the part of its body corresponding to the spot touched by her! Whilst babies may be born with birth marks, there is no truth in this belief.

Care of the teeth

Many people only go to the dentist when they experience toothache, but regular checks are essential in order to maintain good, sound teeth. These may start to decay during pregnancy and deteriorate at a much faster rate than normally, so extra care is necessary.

A balanced diet helps to maintain sound teeth, not only of the mother but also of the baby, whose teeth begin to be formed after the first three months of pregnancy. If too many starchy and sweet foods are eaten, these can damage the baby's teeth.

Keeping fit

Pregnancy is not an illness and many expectant mothers continue to be active, unless for some special reason the doctor advises otherwise. Any sport that the mother has always done regularly can also be continued. It is not advisable, however, to take up a new sport during pregnancy.

Standing, sitting and lifting increase the strain on the body, and ways of doing these are demonstrated at antenatal clinics.

Over-tiredness is best avoided, and the father of the child is able to show his love and attention by helping to do the heavy parts of the housework. If the couple live in an extended family there are usually others around to help; or if the couple is able to afford it, someone is paid to help with the housework.

Sleep

Good sound sleep at night helps the mother to relax, and where possible, short naps during the day help to build up her energy.

Clothes

The pregnant mother may have some favourite clothes which she would like to continue wearing, but squeezing her body into clothes which are definitely too small can be uncomfortable and make her look untidy. Comfortable clothes that hang from the shoulder are much better for her, as are trousers and skirts with expanding waistbands, or dungarees. Comfortable and well-fitting shoes are recommended, since the normal balance of the body is affected by the extra weight; high heels are best avoided.

SOME DANGERS OF PREGNANCY

Usually, pregnancy causes no problems to mother or child, especially in countries where improved medical knowledge and proper antenatal care can help to reduce many of the dangers. However some still exist:

Rubella (German measles)

During the first three months of pregnancy, the danger of malformation of the foetus is greatest. It can be very dangerous if the mother suffers from rubella at this time since serious damage can be done to the baby's brain, sight, hearing or heart. Rubella is caused by a virus and is very infectious. The symptoms can be so mild that very often they go unnoticed. They are a mild pink rash on the face and chest and may be accompanied by a slight fever, swollen glands, and adults may suffer from pains in the joints. The rash may last for only a few hours or for a few days. The best possible protection against the disease is vaccination, which is usually given to girls between the ages of 11 and 14. Under no circumstances should a woman be vaccinated while she is pregnant – she must in fact be vaccinated at least three months before she plans to get pregnant.

Before the rubella vaccine was discovered or used in large-scale vaccination programmes, many children were born with defects (especially hearing loss) to mothers who did not realise they had contracted rubella. All girls and young women are advised to be vaccinated against the disease.

Miscarriage

Sometimes, due to illness or accident or malfunctioning of the ovaries, pregnancy comes to an end by a spontaneous expulsion of the embryo or foetus from the uterus during the first three months. There are times when an abortion may be induced professionally, on medical grounds, if it is in the interest of the mother's health. When the embryo or foetus leaves the mother's body it is described as a miscarriage.

Ectopic pregnancy

In some instances, the fertilised ovum never reaches the womb but stays in one of the Fallopian tubes. This is known as an **ectopic** pregnancy (ectopic means 'in an abnormal place'). In the course of time there is a rupture which causes severe **haemorrhaging** (bleeding) in the abdominal cavity. This condition requires immediate surgery.

Drugs

Towards the end of the 1950s and the early 1960s, thousands of babies were born with terrible deformities; several had no arms, no legs, or tiny limbs resembling flippers. The cause was due to the drug thalidomide which was prescribed for expectant mothers during the fourth to seventh weeks of pregnancy who were finding difficulty in sleeping.

Other drugs can be harmful at different stages of pregnancy. They may damage the ovum before fertilisation, the embryo during the first three months, or the foetus in the middle three months, or have harmful effects on the placenta. Doctors are now therefore very careful about prescribing drugs at this time.

Fortunately most of the drugs required for illnesses such as asthma or heart disease are not harmful to the foetus. But the very tragic cases of the thalidomide malformations showed that there can never be too much care when taking drugs, especially new ones, during pregnancy.

On no account should drugs prescribed for others be taken, no matter how good they are recommended to be.

Alcohol

Just as the food which the mother eats reaches the baby and affects development, so does alcohol. This is a drug, and if the pregnant mother drinks heavily it might cause harm to the foetus.

Smoking

It has been observed from careful studies that babies born to women who smoke during pregnancy are smaller, weaker and slower to develop, so it is advisable for pregnant women to avoid smoking. Women smokers are also more liable to have premature babies.

Hard drugs

These are drugs that are used illegally, such as heroin, cocaine, LSD, amphetamines (stimulants) and barbiturates (sedatives). The user becomes addicted, in other words becomes physically and mentally dependent on the drug. This will probably mean two things: one, the user won't be able to manage day-to-day life without taking the drug and two, won't be able to face the idea of life without the drug.

Hard drugs seriously damage the user's health. In addition the user tends to have no appetite for food and pays little attention to the need for a balanced healthy diet. If the user is a pregnant woman, then this is not good news for the baby. But even worse, just as with alcohol and cigarettes, drugs pass through the mother's bloodstream into the baby's. A baby born to a drug addict will be an addict as well, and will have to be weaned off the drug. Just like an adult, the baby will suffer from withdrawal symptoms.

NAMING THE CHILD

Parents who look forward to a baby very often spend a great deal of time discussing a name. Sometimes this can be the source of argument and disagreement, when one parent insists on choosing a name which the other dislikes. Some parents, in the attempt to give an uncommon name to their child, may choose one that will be a source of embarrassment when the child grows up.

Parents make their choices of names for many different reasons. Some may select names of relatives, or the first boy in the family may be given the father's name and called 'Junior'. Sometimes children, as they grow older, object to this, especially when relatives and others expect them to resemble their fathers in every way. The Bible, novels, movie stars and favourite politicians or their children are other sources of names. Care should be taken in selecting the child's name, as the child is going to grow up and has to carry it all through school life; if the name is strange or the initials are uncomplimentary, such as W. C. or A. S. S., the child may be teased mercilessly by schoolmates. Fortunately, it is possible for persons with names they dislike to change them legally.

Every individual thinks of himself/herself by name, and if it is one that is liked it is a pleasure to carry it.

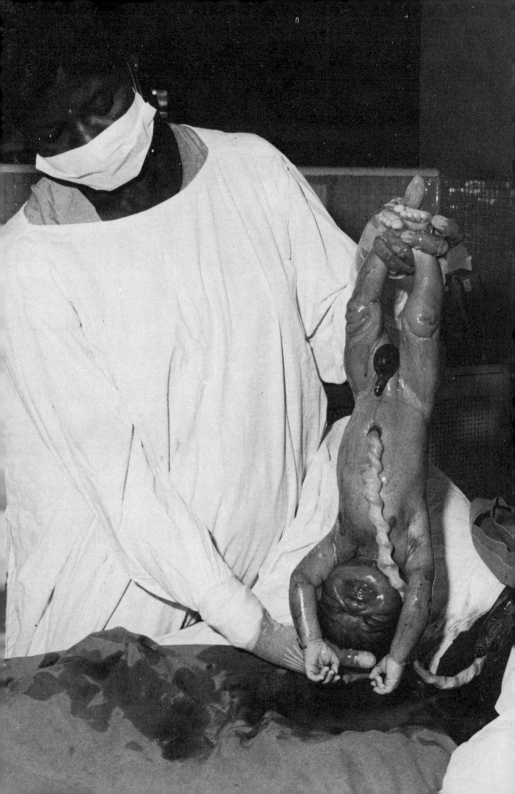

6 Birth of a baby

CONFINEMENT

When the expectant mother goes to bed for the birth of her baby, this is called the **confinement** or 'lying in'. The term 'lying in' is the one more commonly used in the Caribbean. This may take place at home, in hospital, or, in some countries, in a private nursing home. Formerly, most mothers were confined at home and going to hospital was only necessary if there were complications. Nowadays, mothers are advised to go to hospital when having their first baby in case there are any serious difficulties.

There are instances when the baby arrives earlier than expected and many a taxi driver or passer-by has helped at these emergency deliveries! There are also times when mothers have been alone when their baby was about to be born and they have coped with their own delivery. Some of these mothers proudly relate how they managed at the time without even thinking of the possible dangers of this self-help. Fortunately, most such births have been uncomplicated. But more often than not the signs of labour are noticed early and if the mother has been attending the antenatal clinic regularly and remembers all that has been discussed, she avoids anxious moments for herself and others, and ensures a safe delivery of the baby.

LABOUR

The word indicates that the mother must 'work' at bringing her baby into the world.

Signs of the onset of labour
- The abdomen tightens at regular intervals, caused by the contractions of the uterus.
- Bursting of the 'bag of membranes' or **waters** which surround the baby.
- The slight discharge of a blood-stained liquid called the **show**. This is the coming away of the mucous plug which has been protecting the base of the uterus.

HOW HUMAN LIFE BEGINS

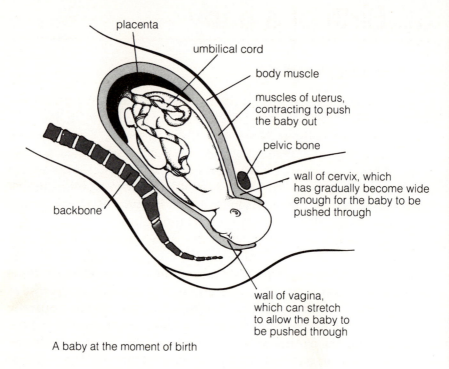

A baby at the moment of birth

Labour takes places in three distinct stages:

Stage 1 is when the mother experiences regular contractions to open up the neck of the uterus, the cervix. This is usually the longest stage of labour.

Stage 2 is when the contractions push the head of the baby gradually and slowly down the vagina to be delivered through the vaginal entrance. This is helped by the 'pushing' of the mother. Once the baby's head becomes visible at the opening, it is described as **crowning**. The baby is then gently eased out by the midwife or doctor. The umbilical cord is then tied and cut. This is the end of the second stage. Sometimes, in order to help the delivery of the baby's head, a little extra room is needed, and a small incision is made at the lower end of the birth canal. This is called an **episiotomy**. After delivery, this is carefully stitched and heals in a few weeks.

Stage 3 is the delivery of the placenta or 'afterbirth'.

Length of labour

The length of labour varies from woman to woman. It may be a few hours, many hours or a few days. Sometimes the contractions stop and restart in their own time, but if the time is too long, there is the danger of the baby suffocating from lack of oxygen. The doctor may induce labour by the injection of a substance to bring on the contractions.

Pain relief during labour

At first the contractions may occur at intervals of twenty minutes, but later they come more frequently. Pain or discomfort is usually experienced with each contraction. It varies from woman to woman. Some may prefer a painless labour and, if available, choose to have an injection (an **epidural**) which causes loss of feeling in the lower part of the body. Others prefer to have an injection which relieves some of the pain during contractions, but which wears off in time for the second stage of the delivery when they can push. Others choose to bear the pain knowing that the uterus is working normally.

COMPLICATED DELIVERIES

Usually, if the baby is in the right position, and the contractions are occurring regularly and strongly, the delivery will be normal. But sometimes complications happen:

Forceps delivery

If the contractions are not resumed sufficiently quickly or are not strong enough in the second stage, the baby may begin to turn blue from lack of oxygen, and the doctor may apply forceps (which are surgical pincers used for lifting) to the sides of the head and *gently* pull the baby through.

Caesarean section

If the labour is exceptionally long and the doctor fears for the baby's safety, or if the mother is physically unable to go through a normal labour, an operation is performed. A small cut is made in the lower abdomen and an opening just large enough for the removal of the baby is made in the uterus. The operation is so called for it is believed that Julius Caesar, the great Roman emperor, was delivered in this way.

Breech delivery

There are times when the baby does not present itself head downwards, but the buttocks or feet show first. This is known as a **breech** delivery. The doctor or trained midwife may be able to turn the baby so that its head is downwards, but if this is not possible, doctors and midwives, using all their experience, may deliver the baby without any harm to it. If no trained help is available there is the danger of suffocation if the baby remains in the breech position for any length of time.

THE MOMENT OF BIRTH

As the baby leaves its mother's body, the first breath is taken with a cry. In the past, the midwife would hold the baby by its feet and slap it sharply if its cry was not quick in coming. This practice is no longer followed; the baby is gently handled. The doctor or midwife who is present at the birth makes a thorough examination for any physical defects, and notes weight and measurement. If the weight is below 2.5 kilos (5½ lbs) the baby is placed in an incubator because it has insufficient body fat and sweat glands to maintain proper body heat. The normal baby is presented to its mother (or parents if father is with her), and the mother holds her baby for the first time.

THE AFTERBIRTH

Between 10 and 30 minutes after the baby is delivered, the placenta or afterbirth is expelled and the birth is complete. An interesting old custom in the folk culture of African slaves in the Caribbean was for the mother to guard the navel string carefully and, after three days to a year from the time of birth, to bury it in the ground and plant a young tree over the spot, which henceforth became the property of the child and was called his 'navel-string tree'. Although the custom is long discontinued among the Afro-Caribbean population, if an individual wants to emphasise that he belongs to a particular place he will say: 'My navel-string was buried there.'

MOTHER'S REACTION TO BIRTH OF BABY

She may be excited and thrilled, or disappointed, but she is usually exhausted.

The first question a mother usually asks is 'Is it all right?' followed by: 'What is it?' Satisfied that the baby is normal, and being very tired and relieved, she will put the baby to the breast, and give him his first feed. She will probably then eat something herself. If the mother is in good health, she is up and out of bed in a few days.

FATHERS AT THE BIRTH

More and more hospitals in western countries, including the Caribbean, encourage fathers to be present at the birth of their babies. Their presence helps to reassure mothers of support, and emphasises the partnership of bringing a new human being into the world. Fathers, too, experience a sense of involvement with the child from its early days. Formerly, fathers waited anxiously outside the room or paced the corridors of the hospital, many smoking endlessly and trying to control their anxiety.

Young single mothers who experience childbirth without the support of the father of their child or any close relative, can feel very lonely and rejected, and some of them desert the baby and leave the hospital without giving an address or any trace of their whereabouts.

THE NEWBORN BABY

The full-term baby

The average newborn baby weighs between three and four kilos and is about 50 centimetres long. On the average, girls are smaller than boys at birth. The newborn baby's head looks much too large for its body. The bones of the head are not fully hardened, but do so gradually. On the top of the baby's head there is a soft spot where the bones have not yet grown together. This spot is called the **anterior fontanelle**, commonly known as the 'mole'! It is covered by a thick membrane and closes gradually in about 12 to 18 months. There is another spot at the back of the head which, if not closed at the time of birth, does so by the time the baby is two months old. Mothers are reassured there is no cause for alarm about these spots, as they are well protected by membrane.

The newborn baby is able to cry, but there are no tears at this stage. The pupils of the eyes react to light, but the eyes are not able to focus. Soon after birth the baby is hungry and will suck if put to the breast. Sucking is a reflex action and is present at birth. Because the muscles are not yet developed, the baby is unable to raise its head or hold it up, therefore the neck and head must be supported when held.

The low birth-weight baby

If a baby is more than two weeks early and weighs less than 2.5 kilos, it is considered a low birth-weight baby. It is immediately placed in an incubator because there is not sufficient body fat and sweat glands to maintain proper body heat. Extra oxygen is also provided.

If the baby is born at home, he may be warmly wrapped and taken to hospital, but low birth-weight babies have been known to survive at home, kept in a very warm box lined with blankets and properly covered hot-water bottles.

When the low birth-weight baby is kept in the incubator at hospital, parents can be very disappointed when mother goes home alone. Hospitals encourage them to visit regularly and the mother is permitted to help with the feeding. This is important to help her to get used to caring and to begin the relationship between herself and baby. The baby is not strong enough to suck for himself so the mother expresses milk from her breasts and feeds this to the baby from a dropper. If the mother is unable to produce enough milk, then a specially prepared formula is fed to the baby in the same way.

The low birth-weight baby develops similarly to the full-term baby but may be slower in the various stages of development such as sitting, standing, walking, talking. If the mother has any anxieties she can visit the clinic and discuss problems with the health visitor. Parents are encouraged not to over-protect the child as it grows up, nor excuse undesirable behaviour on the grounds of his prematurity.

AFTER THE BIRTH

The mother has to adjust to her new life and is usually visited by the health visitor regularly during the first few weeks. The health visitor checks on her adjustment to the baby and on the baby's development. Six weeks after the birth, mother visits the doctor for the post-natal examination.

Post-natal exercises

The mother is advised to practise a few simple post-natal exercises in order to tone up the muscles of the abdomen, and help her figure to return to normal. She is encouraged to continue taking good care of herself by eating a balanced diet, and one that is not too highly seasoned as this may upset the baby's tummy if she is breastfeeding.

'The blues'

Some women go through a period of feeling emotionally low and depressed after the birth of their babies. The period may be short, and the feelings slight or, in some instances, fairly severe. If the mother confides that she is ambivalent towards the baby (sometimes feels love, sometimes indifference), there is need for reassurance that many other mothers have similar feelings in the early stages of adjustment to the new routine.

The young mother who has the support of the father of the child and close relatives around to help and with whom she may talk, gradually overcomes these depressed feelings. Others who may not have the support at home find it helpful to attend mother and baby clinics where they are able to meet and discuss their feelings and anxieties with nurses and other mothers.

The father, too, may be feeling 'blue', a little resentful of all the time and attention paid to the baby, or anxious about the extra responsibility for a new member of the family. If mother and father are able to communicate and discuss their feelings, this very often helps and the 'blues' gradually go away.

In some cases the mother may lose her ability to cope with day-to-day living and she may reject the baby, refusing to feed or respond to it in any way. This is a more serious condition, known as **post-partem depression** and medical help should be sought immediately.

THE BIRTH CERTIFICATE

It is required by law that every birth is registered with the local Registrar of Births.

Having a name for the baby is important, as this makes for an accurate record on the birth certificate. Both parents' names should also be recorded. In some instances when the couple are unmarried it used to be the practice to record only the mother's name, but as long as the father accepts paternity of the child his name is accepted at registration.

The birth certificate is important as throughout later life it is required proof of age on such occasions as entering school, getting married, applying for a passport and so on.

THE NEW MEMBER OF THE FAMILY

Once all the formalities connected with the birth of a baby are completed, the parents are ready to settle down with the routine everyday care of the new member of the family.

BIRTH OF A BABY

BARBADOS

Form P
(Section 34(1))

Vital Statistics Registration Act, 1980

BIRTH CERTIFICATE

Registration Number	8731
When born	3rd October 1985
Name	Marcia Jean Norville
Sex	Female
Name and Surname of Father	Elroy Emmerton Norville
Name and Maiden Name of Mother	Gloria Isabel Norville formerly Gill
Residence of Father	Pine Housing Area, St. Michael
Residence of Mother	Pine Housing Area, St. Michael
Occupation of Father	—
Occupation of Mother	—
Date Registered	21st January 1959
Name and Abode of Informant	Elroy E. Norville Pine Housing Area, St. Michael
National Registration Number	590103-0162

I hereby certify that the above particulars have been compiled from the registration of the birth of the person under reference.

Dated the 23rd day of October 1985

....
Registrar of the Supreme Court.

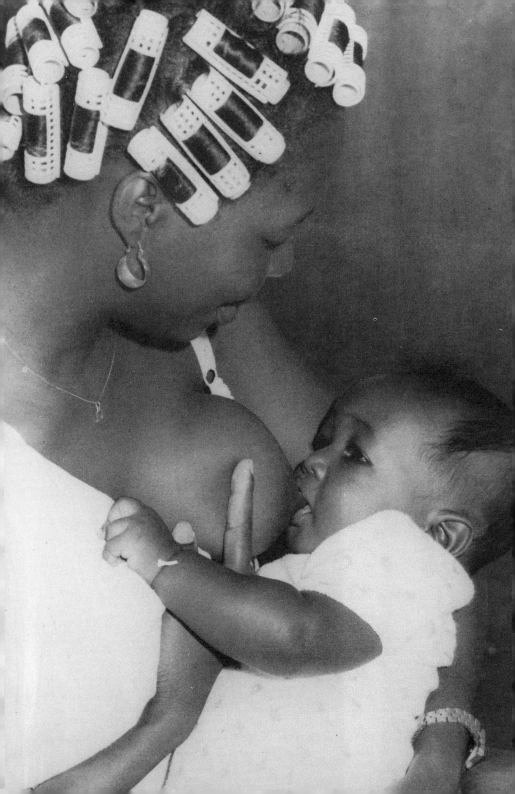

PART THREE: THE EARLY YEARS

7 The physical care of the baby

BREASTFEEDING

Nature provides the perfect food for the baby in the form of mother's milk. If the mother attends the antenatal clinic before pregnancy she will receive advice on the best form of diet to ensure an ample supply of milk. If necessary, the doctor will advise a supplement to her normal diet. She will also be advised on the proper care of the breasts.

When the baby is born, the mother should put the baby to the breast as soon as possible. Babies are born knowing how to suck, though they may need a little help at first in finding the nipple. When the baby's cheek touches the breast the baby will immediately root around, and the mother, with the first and second fingers, can gently guide the nipple into the baby's mouth. The mother should let the baby suck on each breast for 3–4 minutes. What the baby is taking in is not yet milk but a thick, yellowish fluid called **colostrum**. This

BREAST FEEDING
birth to 12 months

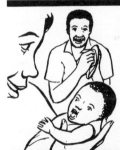

When you are breastfeeding your baby, you should be contented.

This is important because any kind of worrying can slow down your flow of milk. So before feeding your baby, try to have a drink—like fruit juice or water. It will help you to relax. This is also where father can lend a hand, by helping with the housework or with the family, so you can relax and your baby can get the best from the breast.

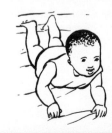

Breastmilk is good for your baby: Your breastmilk ALONE supplies all the food your baby needs for the first *four months* of life. Breastmilk is so good that your baby's body uses it all up to grow strong and healthy. This is why your breastfed baby sometimes does not pass a stool every day. Your breastmilk also helps to protect your baby from vomiting and running belly, polio and measles.

THE EARLY YEARS

fluid – colostrum – provides the perfect nourishment for the baby until the mother's milk 'comes in'. The baby's sucking stimulates the breasts, and in a couple of days the milk, thin and of a bluish colour, begins to flow.

> Remember:– your breastmilk does not cost you any money
>
> – your breastmilk is clean and always ready when your baby needs it
>
> – your breastmilk protects your baby from many germs and diseases
>
> YOUR BREAST IS BEST

In the first days of breastfeeding there may be some problems. The baby may not be too eager to feed, or the nipples may get sore, but as long as mother and baby are in good health and the mother wants to breastfeed the baby, with persistence a comfortable pattern will emerge.

The advantages of breast milk

1 Breast milk contains the required food substances in the correct proportions.

2 It is at the correct temperature.

3 It is clean and pure, provided the mother's personal hygiene is good and the breasts kept clean.

4 It is easily digestible and the baby is less likely to be constipated.

5 It helps to protect the baby from illnesses, as the mother passes on her immunity to disease.

6 There is no time wasted in preparation, so it is ready on demand.

7 It is cheaper than prepared food.

8 Feeding the baby from the breasts helps in the development of a close mother-and-child relationship.

THE PHYSICAL CARE OF THE BABY

Position for breastfeeding

To feed the baby, mother should sit and hold the baby comfortably. She should hold the top of her breast away from the baby's nose so that there is no interference with its breathing. The baby's hands should be free so that the breast may be held. As this is the time when mother and child get to know each other, it is a good idea for the mother to look at the child and hold her face in a position where it may be clearly seen.

Length of feeding time

Not only does sucking give the baby food, warmth and comfort, but it also stimulates milk production. Between 20 and 30 minutes seems to be the usual length of time for any one feed. At each feed the total time should be divided between the two breasts. The one offered first is usually more thoroughly emptied and therefore takes a longer time to be refilled. For this reason, each new feed should begin with the breast which had been offered second in the previous feed.

Problems of breastfeeding

Some mothers may be disappointed that they fail to produce enough milk to satisfy their babies, or that the babies refuse the breast. Being under emotional strain, or being overtired or overexcited can cause a reduction in the quantity of milk that is produced. Mothers who are breastfeeding need adequate rest and sleep, moderate exercise and they should try to keep their emotions on even keel. It is useful if fathers assist as much as possible in and around the house, and show love and affection in order to help in promoting a feeling of security and happiness in the home. If there are worries about financial or other problems, discussing possible solutions with a close relative or friend, a social worker or the family doctor can be helpful.

BOTTLE FEEDING

If for any reason a mother is unable to breastfeed her baby, she can satisfactorily bottle feed. As long as the mother or father take time, the baby thrives from a feeling of comfort and warmth as much as from the actual food, and feeding is a time of closeness and enjoyment for parent and child. One advantage of bottle feeding is that the father may also participate and so begin at an early stage to feel involved in caring. Father and child begin to know one another.

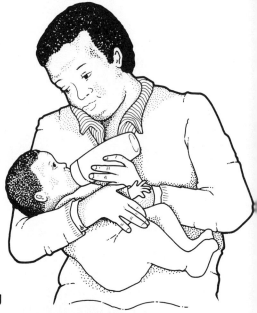

Position for bottle feeding

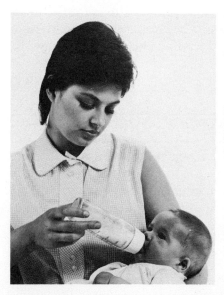
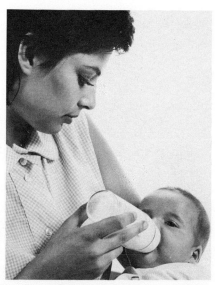

The bottle should be held so that its neck is always full of milk, otherwise the baby will swallow air and might get colic

Whoever is feeding the baby needs to sit comfortably and to be relaxed, holding the baby in a fairly upright position. The bottle should be held so that its neck is always filled with milk – this prevents the baby having to draw on the teat for too long a time, thereby taking in too much air. Whatever the circumstances, the feed should not be rushed. The bottle propped up on a pillow may save the mother or father time, but it is dangerous as the baby may take in too much food at a time and may choke, or the bottle may shift from its position and the feed may go into her nostrils.

Sterilisation

In the preparation of the feed all the utensils must be spotlessly clean, and the hands, nails and clothes of the person must also be clean. These two rules are important because a baby can be easily infected through food prepared in insanitary conditions. Infection may range from tummy upset to gastro-enteritis, which in its severe form can lead to death.

Everything used in the preparation of the feed must be kept covered from dust and flies. The following items are necessary:

- several bottles and teats
- a measuring spoon and knife for levelling the measure
- clean towels for covering
- cleaning brush
- a steriliser: it is not necessary to have one like that used in hospitals and clinics; it can be a large heavy pot in which nothing else is cooked.

To sterilise bottles and teats, teats are placed in a large screw-top jar with holes in the lid. This and the bottles are then boiled in a pot for about 15 minutes. Alternatively, there are commercial solutions available which are equally effective if the instructions are carefully followed.

Mixing the feed

The instructions given with the particular brand of food must be carefully read and followed.

- The hole in the teat must be the right size for the baby. The hole should be larger for babies who take their feed slowly and smaller for quick feeders. A small hole can be enlarged by plunging a red-hot needle (a cold one will not do) into the teat until the hole is the correct size. if the hole is too big the milk will come out too quickly and the baby could choke. If the hole is too small the baby will suck in air, which will give him wind

- The feed should be the same temperature as body temperature. Before feeding the baby the temperature should be tested by squirting some of the milk on the inside of the wrist as this is sensitive to heat.

- A bottle of feed should not be kept warm for very long after being made, as germs develop very quickly in warm milk.

- After every feed it is essential to wash the bottle thoroughly, first in cold water and then with hot water and a brush, in order to remove every trace of milk; the teat should be turned inside out and cleaned under running water. If any of the milk is stuck, the teat may be rubbed with salt. Bottle and teat must then be sterilised.

- It is best to mix each feed at the time it is wanted, but if there is a refrigerator in the house several feeds can be made, cooled quickly, and stored there. At feeding time the bottle should be placed in warm water and brought to body temperature before being given to the baby.

- Older children or adults should not drink from the baby's bottle as it may become infected.

Quantity of food

The quantity of food given depends very much on the size of the baby. A small baby will need feeding more often and will take less than a big baby. On no account should the baby be forced to take more than he needs. It is a good idea for the mother to keep a record of how much is taken and how often the baby cries from hunger, as this helps the health visitor or clinic nurse to advise on the amount suitable for that particular baby. In this way under- or overfeeding can be avoided. Regular attendance at a clinic where the baby's weight is checked is a good way of making sure that she is receiving sufficient food.

THE PHYSICAL CARE OF THE BABY

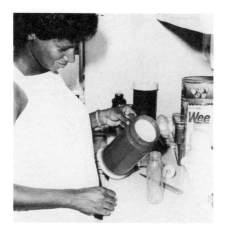

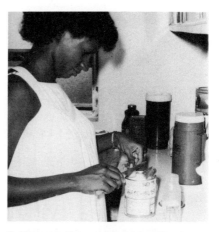

1 First wash your hands. Check pack for how much feed and water is needed. Then measure the correct amount of previously boiled water (cooled to 50°C) into a wide-necked feeding bottle.

2 Measure the powder using the scoop provided. Level off the powder using the back of a knife, without pressing it down.

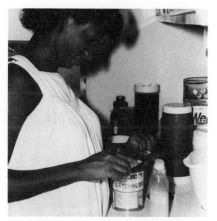

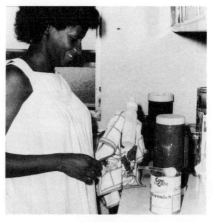

3 Add the correct number of scoops to the powder in the bottle.

4 Place cap on bottle and shake gently until feed is mixed. Then cool feed to the required temperature for your baby by shaking the bottle under the cold tap. Test by shaking a few drops on the inside of your wrist – it should feel comfortably warm.

Feeding patterns

One baby may take all the food at once whilst another may doze and then begin again. Eventually, when satisfied and contented, sleep follows. If the baby does not take all of the food, mother need not become too anxious as long as there are no signs of illness and the baby appears happy and interested in her surroundings.

TIMES FOR FEEDING

Because there are differences in the amount each baby needs, there should be no hard and fast rule for feeding times. It is no good leaving a baby to cry for several minutes because there must be strict feeding by the clock. On the other hand, if she cries too quickly (about half-an-hour after a feed), the reasons should be carefully investigated before feeding again. It may be that there is something wrong: she may be suffering from indigestion or colic; or the diaper needs to be changed.

BURPING THE BABY

Burping is the term used for helping to get rid of the air swallowed whilst feeding. It is usual to do this at the end of the feed; but there are times when it may be necessary to do this during the feed if she slows down and appears to lose interest.

One of the following three ways of burping the baby may be used:

1 The baby is held with her abdomen resting against the shoulder. She is gently rubbed and patted. Hard slapping is not necessary.

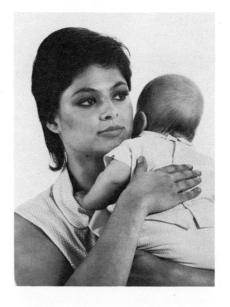

The baby is held with his abdomen resting against the shoulder. He is gently rubbed and patted

THE PHYSICAL CARE OF THE BABY

2 The baby may be placed face downwards across the adult's knees and her back patted and rubbed.
3 The baby may be held in a sitting position whilst the back is rubbed and patted.

Even if, after some time, the baby does not burp, it may be that not much air was swallowed and her stomach is comfortable. If the baby appears to be comfortable there is no need to slap her back.

If the baby seems more than usually uncomfortable and cries a great deal while pulling up her legs a doctor should be consulted.

EARLY PROBLEMS

Colic

Colic is thought to be caused by the pain the baby suffers when wind gets blocked in the bowel. The baby frowns, grimaces draws up her legs and cries with high-pitched screams. The behaviour may last for a few minutes until some relief is obtained when wind is passed. The attacks may last for several minutes or for a few hours, and often occur in the early evening. Some babies seem to obtain comfort by sucking while others are relieved by lying on the stomach. If the attacks persist, the doctor may prescribe a medicine to relieve the pain. When the baby is about three months old, colic usually disappears.

Vomiting

All babies bring up some milk after being fed. Sometimes this may happen when they are held up or when the nappy is being changed after a feed. If the baby continuously vomits the entire feed the health visitor or the doctor at the clinic should be consulted as this may be due to a narrow **pylorus** (the opening of the stomach into the small intestine). And this may require surgery. The doctor should also be consulted immediately if there is any blood brought up, or if the vomit is green in colour, which is a sign of infection.

Frequent vomiting can be a cause of poor weight gain in babies. It is important to take the baby regularly to the mother and baby clinic, so that her weight is carefully monitored. There are other reasons for poor weight gain such as : underfeeding; crying for long periods; or being kept overdressed so that there is loss of fluid in perspiration.

As the baby grows, gradually the pace at which weight is gained slows down, and care needs to be taken at this stage not to overfeed as this can easily result in producing an overweight toddler.

BOWEL MOVEMENT

During the first few days of life, the baby's stool is greenish-black, thick and sticky with little or no unpleasant smell. This is called **meconium**. After a few days the colour changes to light yellow and the stool is soft and unformed. Bottle-fed babies have a firmer stool than breastfed babies.

The times of bowel movement vary from baby to baby, but breastfed babies sometimes may not pass a motion for two days. If the stool is of normal colour and soft and there are no cries of discomfort, there is no need to think that the baby is constipated. On the other hand, if the stools are dry and hard and infrequent the nurse at the clinic or the doctor should be consulted. It is not advisable to give the baby any unprescribed laxative.

Diarrhoea

This means that the stools are much looser than normal and much more frequent. The condition may be caused by a bowel infection; when there is also vomiting it is known as gastro-enteritis. The child should be seen by a doctor immediately.

It is stressed by doctors and nurses that the germs responsible for diarrhoea come from contaminated food or utensils. A good standard of hygiene is therefore necessary in the home. Food and bottles must be kept covered from flies in a cool place or refrigerator, and those preparing the food must have a high standard of personal hygiene.

CHANGING THE BABY'S NAPPY

Nappies (or diapers) are very important items. There are four types: those made from special material known as diaper cloth;

THE PHYSICAL CARE OF THE BABY

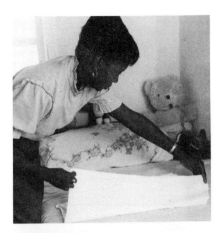
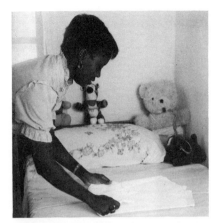
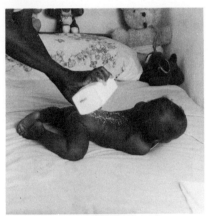
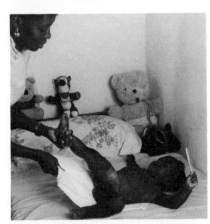
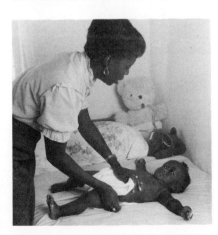
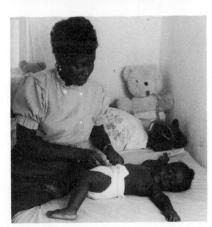

THE EARLY YEARS

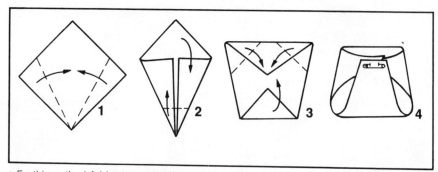

- For this method, fold outer corners inwards to make a kite shape, then fold in top and bottom.

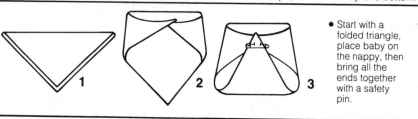

- Start with a folded triangle, place baby on the nappy, then bring all the ends together with a safety pin.

Above are two popular ways of folding cloth nappies. Below, the diagram shows how disposable nappies work.

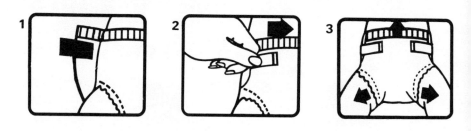

- Remember, always follow the usage instructions.

terry towelling with liners; muslin nappies used especially for very small babies or those with sensitive skins; and disposable ones. Disposable nappies save time and washing but they can be an expensive item as the baby needs to be changed more frequently. Many mothers use a combination of disposables and regular nappies.

When putting nappies on, care should be taken that there is not too much bulk between the legs as this may cause chafing of the skin. When pinning, two fingers should be placed between the baby's skin and the nappy to avoid the risk of pinning the baby's skin.

Care of nappies

If the nappies are properly washed and sterilised they will not hold the germs that start nappy rash. Wet and soiled nappies should never be left lying around, but placed in a covered pail. Soiled ones should be washed off first in the lavatory and then placed in the pail until time for washing. Staining of the nappies can be avoided by washing them as quickly and frequently as possible. Mild soap powder is preferable to harsh detergents. The nappies should first be thoroughly rinsed, and, after drying, folded and stored in a special clean place.

When to change the nappy

When a baby is left in a wet or soiled nappy for any length of time, she soon makes the adult aware of this by crying. Besides being uncomfortable, the soiled nappy can irritate the skin and cause a rash.

Nappy rash

This can be very uncomfortable for the baby. Painful red spots cover the skin all round the nappy area, and the spots may become infected. The rash is caused through the action of germs in the urine and stools when the wet or soiled nappy has been left on for long periods.

To prevent this condition developing, it is important to change the nappy regularly. The baby's bottom should be thoroughly washed with soap and water after soiling and the skin properly dried. If the baby passes stools frequently and the area becomes sore, the skin can be cleaned gently with baby oil instead of soap and water. The health visitor may recommend a suitable cream for the rash. Leaving the nappy off to expose the skin to the air is also helpful for the rash. Plastic and rubber pants should also be left off.

WASHING THE BABY

Bathing

Plenty of time should be allowed in the daily routine so that the bath is unhurried. It may be done either by mother or father. As babies begin to grow, most of them enjoy playing in the water, and bath time is a happy time, with the adult talking and singing to the child, and the baby gurgling back, splashing, kicking or playing with a toy.

Items necessary for the bath
- baby soap and cream
- soft flannel
- cotton wool
- two bath towels
- clean nappy and pin(s)
- clean clothes
- hair brush
- powder
- baby bath at a comfortable working height

THE PHYSICAL CARE OF THE BABY

The following is a recommended bathing routine:

1 Lay everything out for the bath so that there will be no need to leave the baby in the tub to fetch an item from another room: this can be dangerous as the baby might slide and drown.

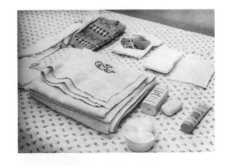

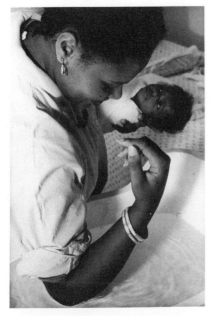

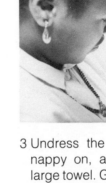

3 Undress the baby leaving the nappy on, and wrap him in a large towel. Gently wash his face with warm water (no soap).

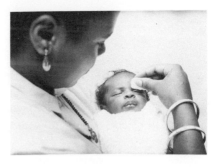

2 Put in cold water first (the bottom of the bath may retain heat if the hot water goes in first, and burn the baby). Add the hot water to bring it to the correct temperature. Test with the elbow to ensure that it is at body temperature.

4 Clean the eyes with cotton wool which has been moistened in cooled boiled water. Use a separate piece for each eye to reduce the risk of infection.

THE EARLY YEARS

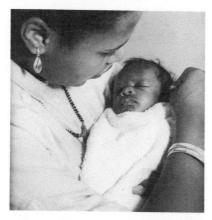

5 Clean the outer ears and the wide part of the nostrils with cooled, boiled water. On no account should the cotton wool be pushed up the baby's nostrils

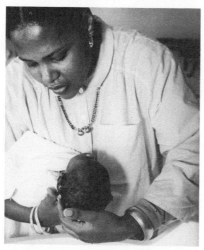

6 Wash the face from the forehead downwards, and, about two or three times a week, wash the baby's head. (The scalp of the baby's head tends to be oily and, if it is not properly cleaned, **cradle cap**, which is a scaly crust, may develop.)

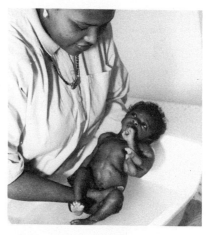

7 Remove the nappy now and place the baby in the bath, firmly supporting him around the shoulders with his head resting on the arm. Gently splash water over him without any hurried movements which may cause alarm.

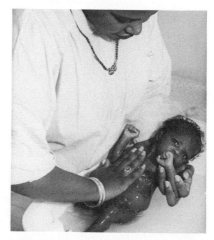

8 Wash the baby over the body with a mild pure soap, paying attention to the folds of the skin under the neck, between the legs and the genital organs.

THE PHYSICAL CARE OF THE BABY

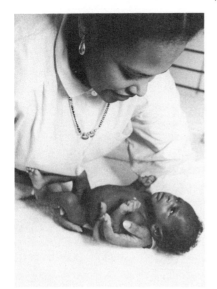

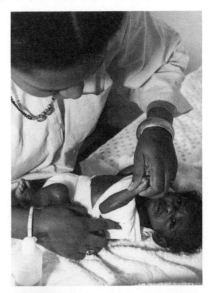

9 Take the baby out of the bath and place him on a dry, warm towel and dry him thoroughly, especially between the folds and creases of the skin.

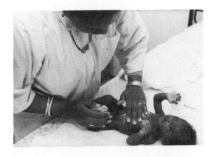

10 Apply talcum powder lightly, as too much may irritate the skin.

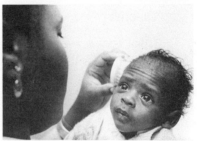

11 Dress the baby making sure she is kept warm, and brush the baby's hair.

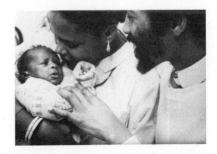

12 He is now ready for a cuddle and a feed.

As babies develop, they enjoy playing more and more in the water. They may like to have water thrown over them, dipped with a cup or gently sprayed from a hand-held spray. There may be crying when the game is stopped, but gently talking and distracting the attention by giving a favourite toy whilst drying her soon helps to restore calm.

Topping and tailing

Topping and tailing is the term used for cleaning the baby without giving a full bath. If the baby has had a bath in the morning, it is a good habit to top and tail her before she is put to bed. As with the bath, everything should be to hand. First of all, the baby's face and neck are washed, dried and powdered, and her vest put on. Then the buttocks are washed, thoroughly dried and powdered, and a clean nappy put on.

Oil bath

If for any reason the doctor thinks it is not wise to bath the baby while she is still very young an oil bath may be recommended. The health visitor or clinic nurse usually shows how to do this, and the instructions should be followed carefully.

CLOTHES

When a woman begins to plan for the arrival of the baby, among the necessary items she prepares are the clothes. These are known as a **layette**. In the layette are found vests, nappies with safety pins, night gowns or chemises, bibs, jackets, bootees, bonnets, waterproof pants.

These may be provided according to the parents' means, but should not be in great quantity as the baby grows fast and will naturally need bigger clothes. Clothing can be very expensive, and sometimes friends and family pass on baby clothes which have been carefully kept. In some families, christening dresses are kept and passed on from child to child.

As the baby grows, additions will be made to the wardrobe according to the parents' budget and tastes, but certain things should be borne in mind when selecting clothes for the young child:

1. The clothes should be made from lightweight material which will not irritate the skin or keep the baby too hot, and which is easily washable.
2. The clothes should be loosely made, making them easy to put on and take off. Back openings tied with tapes prevent the child from having her head stuck in a tight round-neck garment, while the adult pulls and tugs to get it off.
3. If using waterpoof plastic pants, it should be checked that the baby's skin is not sensitive to the material, causing irritation. Also, they should not fit too closely around the thighs.
4. The clothes should provide freedom for normal activity. For example, long dresses will hamper movement when babies begin to move around. Today most of the clothes are unisex and it is sensible to dress girls in rompers and trousers.
5. Stretch-fit clothes do not stretch for ever and these should be replaced as the child grows.
6. Clothes should not be too big as they can be uncomfortable.
7. Clothes for the young child should not have buttons which may be pulled off and put in the mouth, ears or nostrils.

Unsuitable clothes

Sometimes children may be dressed in clothes which well-meaning relatives or friends living in temperate countries such as the USA or Canada or England may send to the Caribbean as presents. The material may be more suitable for those countries than for the tropics, and the sizes may not be the proper ones. The clothes may be very attractive, but may be uncomfortable for the child. If the child's measurements are sent and clothes bought in the summer then there is seldom a problem.

Caring for clothes

The baby's clothes should be washed often, but not with those of older children or adults. A mild soap powder should be used rather than detergents. The clothes should be thoroughly rinsed, dried and ironed, and stored in the baby's cupboard.

TRANSPORTING THE BABY

In different countries different practices are followed in taking the child outdoors after its birth. In some of the Caribbean islands the custom which seems to have been handed down through the African heritage is to take the baby out into the air on the ninth day after its birth. This is an individual matter, and, provided the baby is kept warm she may be taken out as soon as the mother is well. When the mother gives birth in hospital and all is well with her and baby, she may leave after two days with the baby.

It is the practice in the Caribbean for the parent to carry the child cradled in the arms, or in a pram in the early months, and later in a pushchair. Nowadays young parents, mothers and fathers, may be seen carrying the baby in a pouch tied around their chests, leaving the hands free to hold another child or to carry the shopping. The child feels the warmth of the parent's body, and they are both able to see each other's faces and communicate with looks and smiles. Care needs to be taken that the child is comfortable: with the neck and back well supported and the legs not chafed.

Most African women carry their babies on their backs. The baby is lulled asleep by the movements of the adult going about the daily chores, or when awake she can look around at the wonders of the world. The disadvantage is that she is unable to see her mother's face and mother and child are not able to communicate verbally or non-verbally. Most parents select the way that is most comfortable for them and their children.

Selection of prams

The selection of prams and pushchairs depends on the income of the parents. The pram should not be too deep, so preventing the flow of air and making the baby too warm. It should be fitted with efficient brakes. When the baby is left in her pram outdoors, great care needs to be taken to ensure that the brakes are properly engaged and the pram is on level ground, so that there is no danger of it rolling away.

The pushchair should be made of material strong enough to take the child's weight without sagging, and so provide the necessary support for the child's back. It should also have efficient brakes.

THE PHYSICAL CARE OF THE BABY

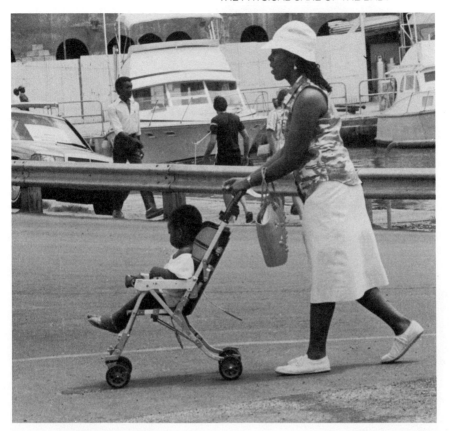

Transport by car

When a young baby is taken by car, the adult holding the baby should sit in the back so that if for any reason the car is brought to a sudden stop there is less risk of injury. If, however, there is no adult passenger to look after the baby, she should be put in a carry-cot or a well-padded box. This can then be secured by covering it with a strong net and tucking the ends down into the seat. A baby who is beginning to turn over and move vigorously should not be transported in this way. The parent should try to enlist the help of an adult or an older child in the family. The safest way of transporting a young child is to have a specially designed baby-seat fitted to the back seat of the car.

All parcels or objects should be removed from the back shelf of the car, as these may fall on the baby if the car stops suddenly.

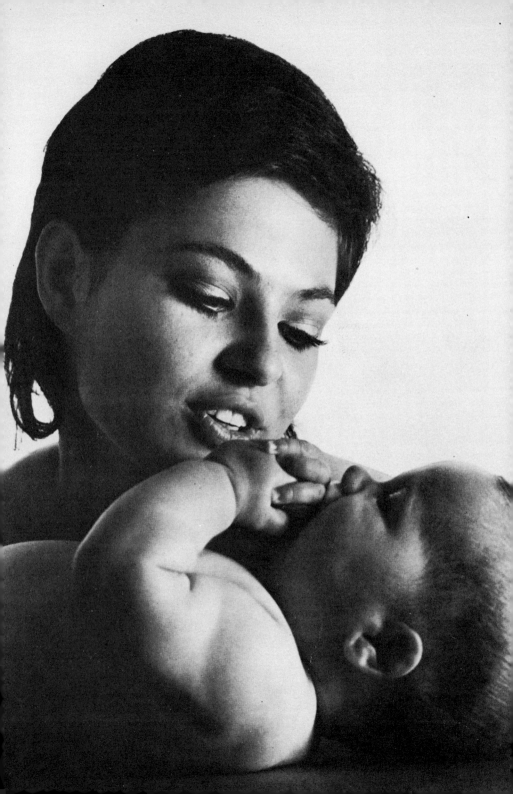

8 Coping with a new baby

THE DAILY ROUTINE

Life in the family undergoes a considerable change on the arrival of a new baby. The major change is that the night's sleep of both mother and father will be interrupted. Some parents take it in turn to get up at nights to feed and change the baby. Each family works out its own patterns for dealing with the change in routine but, in order to make it easy for the mother who has to cope during the day, it is sensible for her to follow a daily routine that not only helps her to get some rest for herself, but also helps the baby to feel safe and secure in the new environment.

The daily routine need not be inflexible. The times for carrying out tasks can vary. It is a framework which should be shaped to suit mother and baby. The following is a suggested routine for a new-born baby:

Daily routine

Morning: about 5.30–6.30 a.m.	Change baby, feed, bring up his wind and, if necessary, change again and put back to sleep.
About 9.30 or 10.00 a.m.	When baby awakens for the second time, bath and playtime, feed, change and put back to sleep.
Afternoon: about 2.30 p.m.	Feed and change. Either allow baby to kick and play a bit, or return to bed to sleep.
Evening: about 5.00–5.30 p.m.	When baby wakes, allow to kick and play a bit, top and tail him, feed, change if necessary and put to bed. If baby sleeps, all well and good, but he may be wakeful. This is perfectly normal, and provides a chance for father to play with his baby.
10.00 p.m.	Feed, change, and settle down for the night.

When the baby is asleep the mother may take some rest and do some of the light housework, making sure not to become overtired. Obviously the baby may not necessarily sleep all the time, and the playing time may be longer between feeds. Some babies may be on a three-hourly feeding time, or mother may be feeding on demand; some babies may sleep through the night, whilst others are very light sleepers and wake frequently. Eventually, a pattern emerges to suit mother and baby.

If the mother is alone, or in a nuclear family, and the father needs to leave home early for work, usually it is she who wakes and comforts the child; but whenever possible the father should be prepared to get up during the night to see to the baby. This sharing helps to maintain a loving relationship between the parents, and taking part in every aspect of caring helps to cement the bond between the child and both parents.

As the baby grows older, he will sleep less and so the routine will include more activity such as playing and taking him out in the fresh air.

It is not necessary to awaken the baby to give a bath or a feed; the times can be adjusted, and if he awakens early there is no need to leave him crying and being miserable until the hour set aside for the activity. The main thing about a daily routine is its flexibility in the interest of the baby.

SLEEP

Babies vary in the amount of sleep they need. On average, babies will sleep 16 hours out of the 24 to start with. Sleepy babies may sleep for 22 hours; wakeful ones may never sleep more than 12 hours. As the baby gets older the hours decrease. The well-fed and comfortably dressed baby who is in good health will sleep in the daylight or in the dark, in spite of the household noises around. Each baby develops its own pattern of sleeping and waking, and, after a time, tends to waken at the same time each day.

By the age of five most children sleep for about 11–12 hours. This is only an average; some seem to need a few more hours, some less. If the baby seems to sleep all day, taking no notice of his surroundings, or if he seems to be awake all night, then this should be discussed with the **paediatrician** (doctor specialising in children's illnesses).

As the child grows older and becomes more interested in his

environment, the less inclination there is to sleep during the day. Very often the child who protests about being put to bed during the afternoon may cry, but will be found sound asleep shortly afterwards, thus indicating that the sleep was needed. If he does not sleep during the day, then an early bedtime will help to give the extra hours.

Aids to sound sleep

1. **The bed:** a baby should have its own cot with a firm safe mattress, covered with a rubber sheet to protect it, and then a sheet of cotton which should be well tucked in to keep it smooth. No pillow is used for the first year. The bars of the cot should not be too wide in case the baby gets its head caught between them. There should be a blanket (lightweight) for covering the baby in cold weather.
2. **Fresh air:** fresh air is good for the baby and, provided there is a safe area near the house such as a front porch or backyard without overhanging trees which may drop fruit suddenly, the child may be put in his pram, well-protected from insects by a net.
3. **Clean baby:** the baby should be clean on being put to bed. If the skin is hot and sticky, this could prevent dropping off to sleep easily.
4. **Clothes:** the sleeping clothes should be roomy and comfortable and changed frequently.

CRYING

A young, normally healthy baby will cry from time to time. It is one way of communicating his needs. If he is properly fed, clean and in a comfortable bed, he will eventually go to sleep contentedly, realising that mother will not pick him up every time. Adults in the family need to appreciate mother's attempts at training, and not pass the baby from hand to hand like a family toy. The mother may show love by bending over the cot, talking and making reassuring noises, drawing attention to mobiles hanging over the cot, or the movement of leaves and branches, if outdoors.

If the baby does not cry, it should not be thought he is a good baby. It may be a sign of some retardation, and a doctor should be consulted.

THE EARLY YEARS

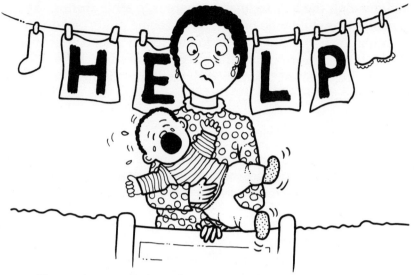

Time, patience and love are fully compensated for

Reasons for crying

A baby may be crying for any of the following reasons:
- **Hunger**: as soon as the baby feels hunger pains he will cry.
- **Discomfort**: the baby may need to have his nappy changed.
- **Tiredness**: the baby may simply be overtired. In this case leave him a few minutes until he falls asleep.
- **Wind**: the baby may still have wind and need to be burped.
- **Loneliness**: the baby may need to be cuddled, or fed for comfort.
- **Wrong temperature**: he may be over- or underdressed.
- **Pain**: the baby may be poorly – medical advice is needed.

The baby's cries should not be ignored. With experience, adults are able to tell fairly accurately what the cries tell; whether it is the cry of hunger or the fretful cry when fighting against sleep, or the sharp piercing cry of pain.

However, if all the baby's needs are met, and crying persists, it may be that there is something seriously wrong. Perhaps an illness is coming on. The adult should avoid getting into a panic, but seek advice from the clinic nurse or doctor.

The use of a dummy

In order to stop a baby crying, some mothers resort to a dummy. Whilst the sucking action may provide some comfort, a dummy is no substitute for the love given by cuddling and talking to the baby. The time spent in doing this is well worth it in helping to make the baby feel secure. The use of a dummy might slow down the child's language development, as the usual gurgling and babbling does not take place.

A dummy that is not clean can be a source of infection which may be one of the causes of gastro-enteritis. Sometimes adults are seen sucking the dummy before giving it to the baby. This is not a desirable habit as the baby has not yet built up immunity to diseases. Dipping the dummy in sweetened juices encourages the taste for sugar which can lead to the early decay of teeth.

Sometimes the baby's crying upsets the young parent, who tries to stop it by vigorous shaking or slapping, which only serves to make the child cry more. If anyone caring for a baby ever feels it is impossible to cope with the crying, instead of slapping or shaking him, they should seek help from a close friend, neighbour or relative, and take the child to the doctor or clinic for a check.

The cause of the crying may not be physical but could be due to unhappiness in the home. The parents should be helped to discuss their feelings toward the baby, especially if one of them is a step-parent. There may be some resentment toward the child. Parents may be worried about personal problems: for example the father may be unemployed and unable to support the family adequately.

If there are no members of the extended family able to help, a social worker may discuss with the parents the advisability of placing the child with foster parents temporarily until their situation improves. In some cases the placement may become permanent.

In the early weeks, both parents tend to feel tired and anxious, and might experience difficulty in adapting to a new lifestyle. But this time is comparatively short in a human being's lifespan, and the time, patience and love is eventually fully compensated for by the joys of parenthood.

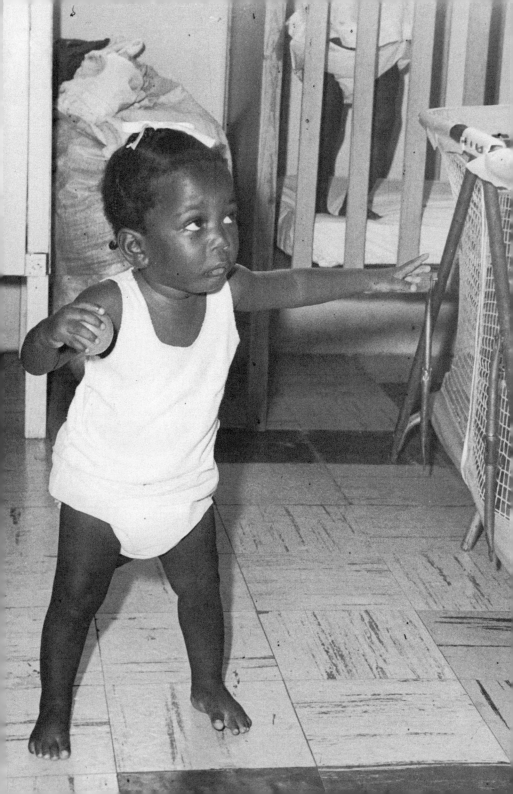

9 The importance of the first years

Whether or not a baby is planned, when it comes into the world it deserves the loving and thoughtful care of both parents. The following chapters suggest ways of caring for the young child, but what no one will be able to help parents do for their babies is to love and enjoy them. The early years of the child's life are the most interesting and most demanding; they are also the most important for laying the foundation for the sort of person the child will become, and for building relationships with the parents who care for her.

The needs of children can be classified into the following categories:

- ♥ **Physical**: this includes the need for food, shelter, clothing, fresh air and exercise.
- ♥ **Emotional**: to be loved, and to love in return; to be secure, that is, to have a feeling of being safe; to be able to trust people and to be free from fear that the adults nearest and dearest will ill-treat or desert her.
- ♥ **Social**: to be in the company of older persons such as parents and other family relatives and friends from whom the ways of the society may be learnt; to play with other children. In the early stages of life small children will play alongside each other, but gradually will appreciate opportunities to share and play as members of a team. From the people in the environment the child will learn language and so increase the ability to communicate.
- ♥ **Intellectual and aesthetic**: to be stimulated to think and to explore the environment; to learn about various materials and their uses; to be encouraged to create, and to be exposed to the works of others through books and other means. The child needs to have her attention drawn to the beauty of nature and so helped to develop an aesthetic sense and an appreciation of the environment. Children who are helped in this way are seldom destructive.
- ♥ **Spiritual**: the child needs to be made aware that most people believe in a supreme Power greater than man, and that people of different faiths call this Power by different names, such as God, Allah, Buddha, and so on. As she grows she has to be helped to be tolerant of others' beliefs and customs.

GROWTH AND DEVELOPMENT

In the normal average baby, growth and development of the body, mind and personality progress in harmony and at a more or less predictable rate. Babies grow much faster in weight than in height. In about five or six months the baby doubles her birth weight, and at one year this is trebled.

However, no two babies develop at the same rate, and no mother or caretaker should expect that the child will achieve an accomplishment at the exact times set out in a baby-care book. These only provide a rough guide. However, development will follow the same general order and pattern, so it is best to observe the order rather than the time. Some children will develop a little faster, some a little slower. When the development is too slow then something is wrong – the child may be deaf, or blind, or mentally retarded, and medical advice should be sought.

Milestones along a road tell us the distances between places; so the various stages in the child's development are commonly called milestones, since they mark various points on the road to maturity.

How a child develops

Each child is born with certain characteristics which develop in a certain way. Conditions in the environment will influence the rate of growth; for example, poor nutrition, severe illness or lack of love and affection tend to stunt physical growth. Other factors which may influence the personality and emotional development of the child may include the position in the family – the first child whose mother may have stayed at home and given her undivided attention is more secure and more outgoing than the second or third child, who may have been left in a day nursery where as much individual attention was not possible. A last child, or one born after a long interval and who is the baby, not only to parents but to brothers and sisters and other relatives in the family, will also develop differently from the others, perhaps by being dependent for a longer period. The only boy in a long line of girls, or vice versa, or an only child, usually tends to receive more attention from parents and relatives, and may develop into a self-centred person, or a very self-assured person.

THE IMPORTANCE OF THE FIRST YEARS

The child who may have suffered from poor health during its early years may be overprotected by members of the family, and this may lead to the individual who expects to be treated gently always, who is timid and who tends to use illnesses as a way of getting out of stressful situations. On the other hand, the individual may develop into a very independent person in an attempt to prove her ability to cope.

The adults who are closest to the child in the early stages of her life will influence attitudes and behaviour to a very large extent. Children observe far more than adults think they do, and just because in their early years they are unable to talk, this does not mean that they do not understand. Far more goes on behind those wide-open eyes than adults believe. It is therefore very important that desirable examples are set, for children learn through imitation.

Individual differences

Each child in some way resembles both parents, but also has her own characteristics which are unique and make her an individual person. Each individual child develops at her own rate in every way. Children from the same parents living in the same house react differently to situations because of this difference. It is not wise to compare children's development. For example, a parent may say of one child 'He is slow, he should be talking; when his sister was his age she was talking.' It is natural to notice these differences, but parents need to be aware that there are many factors which influence the development of children; one such is that girls develop at a faster rate than boys in the early years.

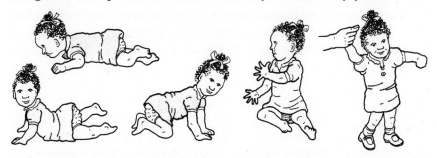

THE EARLY YEARS

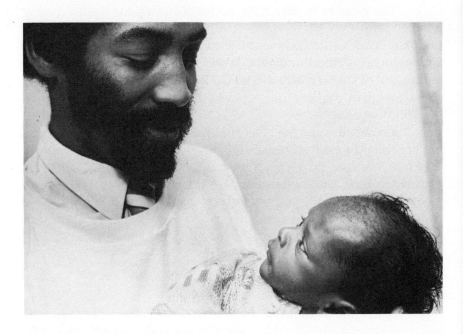

Development in the first year

The following gives the average development rate. Some babies will be slower, others faster. Some babies may learn to crawl early, but walk late. There are no hard and fast rules.

At birth 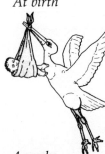 There is very little control over actions. The baby waves her arms and her legs go up and down at the same time, the head wobbles if it is not supported and the eyes have a vacant stare. By the end of the first week a bright light will cause the baby to turn her eyes towards it. She is startled by sudden loud noises, stiffens, screws up her eyes, stretches, and may cry.

4 weeks 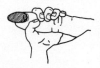 The expression is still vacant, the hands are usually closed, but if a finger is pushed in, she will grasp it. She might stop crying when she hears a human voice. At this stage she cannot distinguish between her parents and other adults.

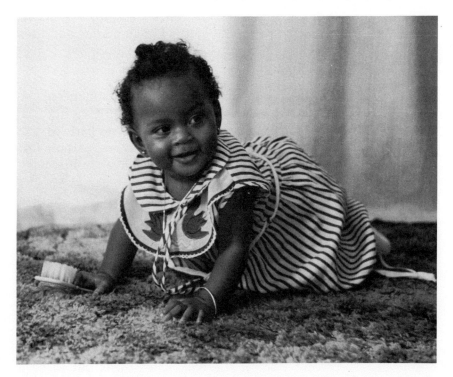

4–8 weeks 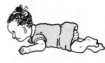	Baby's first smile comes when she hears a voice. When lying on her stomach she is able to lift her chest. She begins to make sounds when lying awake. She coos and gurgles and seems able to recognise her mother's face.
3–4 months 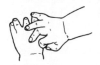	Baby is able to hold her head up as the neck muscles are getting stronger; she moves her head around and takes an interest in the surroundings, she can hold a rattle for a few moments. She begins to discover her body and plays with fingers and toes.
5–6 months	Baby can really laugh and makes all sorts of noises. She will be able to hold her head more erect. She reaches for and grasps an object dangling in front of her: everything goes into her mouth at this stage. She knows her mother's voice and seems to recognise other people. She kicks strongly and can roll

over front to back and back to front. When her hands are held, she braces her shoulders and tries pulling herself up to a sitting position. She can sit propped up with cushions.

7–8 months

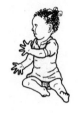

She begins to react differently to strangers; she may stare at an unfamiliar person or turn her face away or scream. This reaction is part of the normal development of a baby. Many parents feel embarrassed when the baby behaves in this way, but this shows the developing ability to tell the difference between mother and other human beings.

9 months

Baby is able to sit without support for a short time; and begins to crawl. She tries pulling to stand and sometimes falls backward, as she is unable to lower herself. She can now use her hands more expertly, splashing in the bath, waving 'bye-bye'. Most babies usually use both hands equally. The use of the right hand usually increases in the second year. If the child later turns out to be a left-hander there should be no attempt to change this as it will be confusing. She is able to babble and make the sounds 'da da' and 'ma ma'. She imitates sounds.

12 months

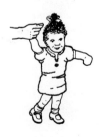

She can now sit for longer and can sit up from lying position. She holds on to furniture and pulls herself up and is able to let herself down. She is able to take steps forward with one or both hands held. At this stage the baby enjoys throwing toys forward and shows pleasure when these are returned. She recognises familiar adults, and is very interested in watching her surroundings. Indeed everything is of great interest. She knows her name and responds to it; 'talks' loudly and with expression as though carrying on a conversation. Simple instructions are understood such as, 'Clap hands'. She knows the use of various objects such as a cup and spoon.

WEANING

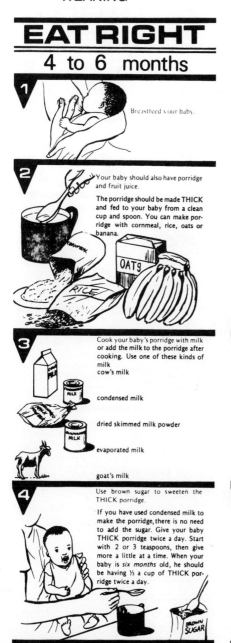

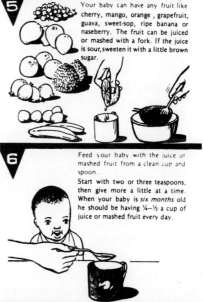

For the first three months the baby is breast fed on milk. Sometimes cooled boiled water is also given. If she is well and progressing normally by this time, semi-solids such as thoroughly cooked cereal, mashed fruit or vegetables may be introduced in small quantities. At first the taste will be strange and she may well refuse to eat it. In this case she should not be forced, but another flavour tried. Given when the baby is hungry, just before the breast or bottle, she will usually take it. Strained fruit juice once a day is also recommended.

From 'Eat Right, 4–6 months', Ministry of Health, Kingston, Jamaica

THE EARLY YEARS

In the Caribbean fruits such as mangoes, cherries, pawpaw and bananas provide adequate vitamins and minerals. It is not necessary to buy expensive imported puréed fruits.

Every mother will decide the best routine for weaning her baby. In the days of our grandparents, mothers breastfed for periods of nine months to a year. They had observed that the longer they breastfed their children, the less chance they had of becoming pregnant. Breastfeeding then was used as a means of birth control.

Recently, since more mothers go out to work, they will breastfeed their babies for shorter periods, perhaps three or four months. Whatever the length of time, weaning should be gradual, with a mug and spoon or a bottle feed being substituted for one feed at a time, until eventually the mug and spoon or bottle is given at every feed.

EAT RIGHT
6 to 12 months

1 Now also give your baby food from the family pot.
Take out the baby's food before you add hot pepper, curry or any other strong seasoning. Mash the food by rubbing it through a clean strainer with a clean spoon.

2 If you are giving your baby fish or meat,
make sure it is cut into very small pieces.

3 You can soften your baby's food with
butter or margarine
milk
a little pot water or gravy.
Always feed your baby from a clean cup and spoon.

From 'Eat Right 6–12 months', Ministry of Health, Kingston, Jamaica

Development in the second year

When the baby passes her first birthday she starts making great strides, and her development is even more varied. The baby learns to walk, to speak recognisable words, to hold and drink from a cup. She can play with toys and spends a lot of her time exploring the environment. Using her newly discovered skill of walking, she can learn to climb, to dance, to balance and to jump. But beware, she can move very quickly and requires constant supervision! Or the baby may be more interested in sitting down and looking at pictures, at drawing or painting, at seeing how one thing fits inside another.

Gradually the baby becomes a toddler, and as she does so may experience frustration or confusion as her new independence clashes with her desire for protection. It is a time when the parent needs a great deal of patience, and love.

THE JOYS OF THE FIRST YEARS

As we have seen, children develop at different rates, depending on their interests and character. Whatever the rate, seeing a child make her first step, or hearing her say her first words is always a joy to the parents and adults in the family. The sheer joy and excitement on the baby's face thrills the adult and compensates for the sacrifices made in the early years of its life.

INDEPENDENCE

As the child grows there will be the urge to be less dependent on adults. Parents and other members of the family will try to provide opportunities and encourage this independence, at the same time setting limits in order that the child may know how far to go. At times, disappointments and frustrations occur when the adult says 'no' to some activity the child wants to do, but very often an alternative can be found.

PHYSICAL HANDICAPS

If parents are observant they will realise at an early stage if the child has any physical handicap such as deafness or blindness. If the child does not hear sounds and the human voice she will not be able to speak. So if the baby lies passive and quiet for too long, not showing any interest in her surroundings as the weeks and months pass, this must not be mistaken for being a 'good baby'. Advice should be sought from the health visitor and a diagnosis and treatment obtained from the paediatrician.

TALKING TO THE BABY

Some mothers have confessed to feeling silly talking to the baby who is unable to answer, but it is essential that the child hears the human voice at an early stage, for this helps in the development of language. When the baby makes babbling and gurgling sounds, adults repeating these sounds not only show their love and affection and interest, but stimulate the child's first words.

Baby talk

Because children are naturally imitative, adults' speech will be imitated and it is important that words are pronounced in the accepted manner of speech. Baby talk or mispronouncing words and using shortened forms of words such as 'bic-bic' for biscuit, should be avoided, as this tends to hamper the child's vocabulary. If the child invents words for certain objects or certain people, then she should be gently told the correct word or name. If she persists in using the 'wrong' words for various objects, she should not be punished and discouraged from talking. The correct word can simply be inserted at appropriate times in the adult's speech, and gradually the child will learn its correct use.

Teeth

Long before the baby's first tooth appears, the 20 **milk teeth** (as the first teeth are called) are fully formed under the gums. On rare occasions a tooth is visible at the time of birth, but normally the teeth start to appear at about the age of six months. This may be earlier or later, depending on the individual rate of development of the child. If, however, no teeth have appeared after twelve months, the doctor's advice should be sought.

All those concerned with the care of pregnant women stress the importance of including foods rich in vitamin D (essential for building bones and teeth) in the diet. So, too, is a balanced diet necessary for the growing baby, if necessary supplemented with vitamin D for the maintenance of the teeth. This vitamin is also known as the sunshine vitamin, and people living in the tropics are fortunate to have it free of cost as it is absorbed from the sunlight through the skin.

THE IMPORTANCE OF THE FIRST YEARS

Pattern of teething

Generally speaking, the teeth appear in the order indicated on the following diagram:

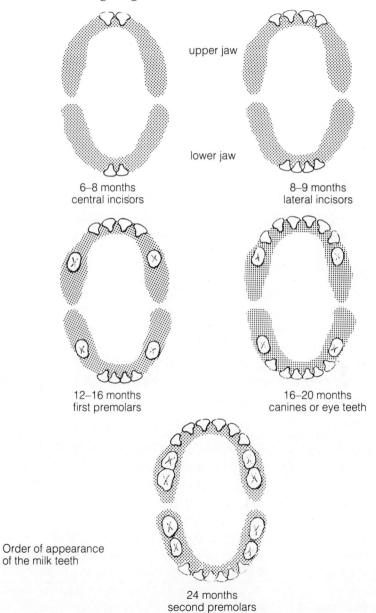

6–8 months
central incisors

8–9 months
lateral incisors

12–16 months
first premolars

16–20 months
canines or eye teeth

Order of appearance
of the milk teeth

24 months
second premolars

Signs of teething

As the teeth begin to come through the gums, it seems as though they tickle or hurt, and there may be some slight or severe discomfort. The baby may begin to bite on objects within reach, including the sides of the cot. (If this is painted, the paint needs to be non-toxic, and the surface of the cot needs to be kept clean.) Dribbling increases and the gums may appear red and slightly hot to the touch. They may be lightly massaged with a clean finger dipped in cool, boiled water. There may be loss of appetite and fretful crying at times.

Teething is not necessarily difficult but if weaning was sudden and the baby is adjusting to being bottle-fed at the same time that teeth appear, she may need some extra attention. If, however, there are signs of illness such as vomiting, a high temperature, or diarrhoea, the baby may have picked up an infection and it is important that the health visitor or doctor sees her at an early stage.

Care of the teeth

The set of 20 milk teeth eventually come through by the middle of the third year. They are very important to the child not only for chewing, but because they help in the proper development of the jaw in preparation for the permanent teeth. If the milk teeth are not properly cared for and cavities develop, the child may chew on one side of the mouth only. If this habit is prolonged an uneven development of the face may be the result.

After feeding, the first teeth may be cleaned by gentle wiping with a piece of sterilised lint. Later a baby's toothbrush may be used. The toddler should be taught how to brush the teeth correctly, the teeth in the upper jaw brushed with a downward motion from the gum, and those in the lower with an upward motion and the molars or jaw teeth brushed across the surface also. The child should be encouraged to take time when cleaning her teeth and to rinse thoroughly to get rid of food particles, especially before going to bed. If the child attends a good nursery school the proper care of the teeth will continue there and so reinforce the parents' teaching at home.

Too many sweets, sweetened drinks, ice creams and jellies can cause decay. If given only moderate amounts the child can be trained to wash her mouth immediately after eating them. This helps to cut down on tooth decay. The toddler develops a taste for sweets only if given them by adults, and the practice of giving a bag of sweets when leaving the child at the playgroup or nursery school is one that should not be encouraged. It is far better to give a fruit, or, best of all, nothing but the parent's love and assurance of being back on time when all the other children are being collected.

The child and the dentist

Unfortunately, many parents do not bother to take their young children to the dentist unless they complain of pain. It is advisable to take the toddler from around the age of three in the company of one or other parent so that she becomes familiar with the routine of examination. This helps to prevent the fear of the dentist that so many people have and encourages taking good care of the teeth. Although the teeth may look sound, only a thorough examination will reveal any cavities, especially in the molars or back teeth.

In some countries there are school dentists specially trained to deal with young children and they help to make the child's first impression of examination and cleaning of the teeth a positive one.

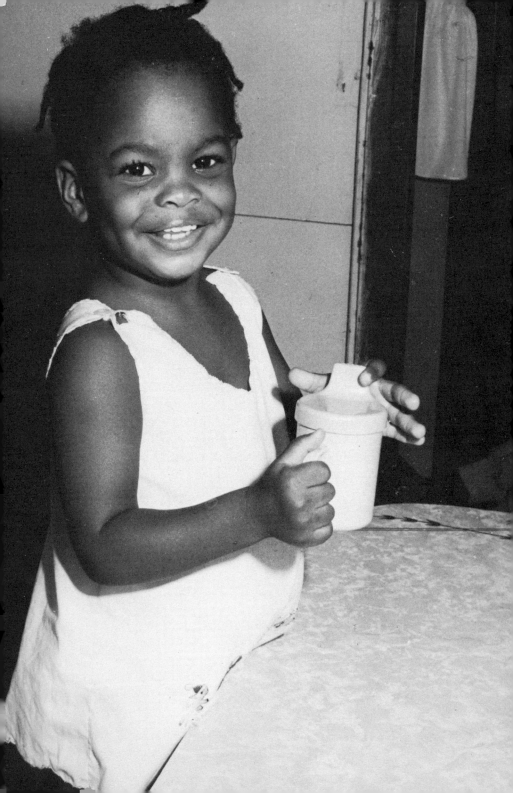

10 Caring for the toddler

The second year of the child's life is one of very rapid growth. Several changes take place in this short time. No longer is there total dependence on adults. The average normal child between the age of 18 months and two years is able to feed himself and move around the house independently. What he wants and how to obtain it is very definite. He recognises his name and responds when called, and has a clear expectation of parents and other family members. He begins to take an interest in life outside the home.

The child who is loved seems able to sense this, and tends to be more confident than the one who is not, and is far more likely to explore the environment. He toddles – that is, walks with short unsteady steps (hence the name 'toddler'), at great speed and therefore needs to be closely supervised and limits need to be set for his safety. For example, the child's hand is held when walking in a busy street or at crossings, but in the safety of a properly enclosed and supervised playground this is not necessary.

CARE OF THE FEET

Because the toddler is now walking and moving around so rapidly, proper care of the feet is important at this stage of development. The flat foot of the baby changes as the soft ligaments begin to mature and arches gradually appear as the feet begin to support the body. Exercise of the bare feet helps and indoors, where the floor is safe, or outdoors, on grassy ground free from stones and jutting-up tree roots, the child is best left without shoes.

When the first shoes are bought the feet should be measured carefully for width and length. They should not be too big with the thought that they will last longer and fit as the feet grow. Blisters on the feet may develop as the shoes slide up and down, and the child may practise clawing the toes in an attempt to keep them on. Shoes should be roomy enough to allow the toes to spread naturally, and they should fit well around the ankle and over the instep. Socks should also be roomy so that the foot is not cramped before fitting into the shoes.

Some parents buy shoes for their young children by measuring the foot with a piece of string, which they then take to the shop to measure the sole of the shoe. This is not the best way of selecting shoes; the child should be taken whenever possible to have shoes fitted, even if it takes a little more time. The measurement should be from the tip of the longest toe to the heel and about half-an-inch should be allowed between the tip of the longest toe and the tip of the shoe.

No two people walk exactly alike and therefore shoes should not be handed down from one child to the next during the stage when the feet are still developing. It is not worth endangering the child's posture and the proper growth of the feet.

The young child grows very rapidly, and this needs to be borne in mind when budgeting the cost of caring for him. It may be wise to save on other items of clothing and spend the extra on providing suitable shoes as the feet develop. Many an adult goes limping through life because they wore faulty shoes in early childhood.

CURIOSITY

Curiosity leads to investigation of most things within sight, and, while fragile and valuable objects should be put away until the child is older, he should be taught that not everything in sight can be touched. This can be done by saying 'no' gently but firmly when an attempt is made at taking an object, and by giving him a toy of his own to play with. Gradually the toddler learns what he may or may not touch.

CHANGE IN PARENT–CHILD RELATIONSHIP

A young child is **asocial** – that is, not caring of others. Through imitation he soon begins to realise what is acceptable within the family and later in the wider society. The baby's way of getting what is needed is to cry; the toddler, on seeing what he wants, frequently grabs and shows his anger if not allowed to do this. Patiently he is taught to ask for things and to say, 'Thank you'.

The toddler who is enjoying the new-found independence frequently says 'No' and refuses to do what he is told. The adult needs to remain calm, although the parent who has to get through a busy day may find it difficult at times to be patient and to wait. But this is a stage through which the child passes. One way of dealing with the child is to physically lift him when he refuses to budge, at the same time explaining why this is being done. For example, 'Yes, it is time to eat.' The child soon learns when it is unreasonable to say 'No'. The toddler begins to understand why things are done the way they are done, and therefore parents should be prepared to give reasons. For example, 'Toys must be put in the box, so that no one will step on them', 'or so that you know where to find them'.

There are times when speaking sharply to the child is necessary. For example, 'Stop' if he is about to run into the street. Usually, from the tone and urgency in the voice, the child obeys immediately! Sometimes a quick slap will stop the child from being hurt. For example, touching a hot iron or poking a finger in the fire. But slapping must not be used continually, as in time this will become meaningless to the child.

SELF-DISCIPLINE

Parents need to be consistent in the way they teach what is acceptable behaviour and what is not, for only in this way will self-discipline develop. Discipline must not be confused with punishment. Self-discipline is the ability to stop oneself from doing what is not acceptable in the home or in the wider community.

PUNISHMENT

Corporal punishment or, as it is commonly called, 'beating' is usually not necessary with a toddler. Even to a small child there are ways of punishing that seem fair and logical; for example, if the toddler draws on the wall instead of on paper provided, taking the pencil away for a while helps to stop this, rather than hitting and scolding. There are some ways that a child should never be punished, for example by withholding food or shutting him in a dark room.

Parents should not make their children afraid of them; explaining and reasoning in the early years helps to build the foundation for trust, mutual respect and love.

EXPRESSING FEELINGS

A toddler who may not be too happy and needs the attention of parents or adults may cry for long periods without any provocation; or may cry for a hurt which appears trivial to the adult. The crying serves to draw attention to unhappiness. There may be a baby in the family and jealousy soon shows itself in this way, or the toddler may have started nursery school and misses home. Very often boys are told 'Men do not cry!' The child is not a man, and why should men not cry? – they are human too!

Children need to be allowed to cry to express their grief or hurt or disappointment, but they also have to be helped to stop crying. This should not be done with threats such as 'If you don't stop crying I will beat you.' Threats only serve to make matters worse and to make the child feel unloved.

If there is a young baby in the family, time and attention need to be given to the toddler; if there is an accident the child should be comforted. We all know how 'kissing it to make it better' works wonders.

Persistent crying may be the advance notice of one of the usual childhood illnesses, and the clinic nurse or doctor should be consulted if in any doubt.

THE TODDLER AND SLEEP

Children vary in the amount of sleep they need, and sometimes the toddler may awaken early and seek their parents' company. A drink of water may be given and after some reassurance that parents are there he goes back to bed. This can be very disturbing to the working parent or parents who may be tired. The child should be encouraged to stay in his bed and not disturb others, and will do so more easily if emotionally secure.

Care should be taken that there is not too much exciting play before bedtime. This tends to make for overtiredness and overstimulation which may interfere with sleep. In some homes where the toddler may share a bed with a brother or sister, the bed should be big enough to ensure that they are comfortable and will not disturb each other. The young child who is continuously deprived of a good night's sleep tends to be irritable and unpleasant during the day.

REFUSING TO GO TO BED

Many parents complain that they find it difficult to get their toddlers to go to bed at a reasonable hour at night. There may be several reasons for this – there might be a great deal of activity in the house, or the parents may be inconsistent, with one parent saying 'Go to bed' and the other saying 'Let the child stay up to watch television'! No wonder then that going to bed becomes a problem. If all adults in the house are consistent, this will help the child to follow a routine. On special occasions, for example a relative arriving late from abroad, the child may be allowed up. If he is not attending nursery school, the extra hours may be made up by sleeping late the next day.

Children must *not* be left alone in a house asleep. They may waken and become very afraid on realising that they are alone. Anything may happen whilst parents are out; one of the dangers is the risk of fire, and many a child has died as a result of a fire which broke out when the parents were out.

Even if this extreme accident should not occur, emotional damage can be done to the child who has been put to sleep believing that parents are there, and awakens needing a drink or the potty, only to find no one there. This can lead to sleeping difficulties, a growing mistrust of adults, and lack of respect for parents' words.

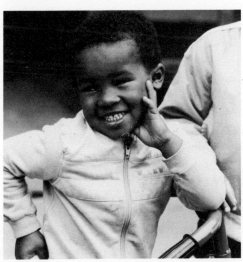

FEEDING THE TODDLER

A malnourished child is an unhappy child who seldom smiles and one who will become ill easily and often. Poor nutrition stunts growth physically, mentally and intellectually.

The importance of a balanced diet

It is essential that the child has a balanced diet. Every day there should be a helping of one of the foods rich in body-building protein, vitamins and minerals. These are found in the following: eggs, fish, meat, peas or lentils, milk, cheese, fresh fruit, leafy green vegetables, bread and cereals. Nibbling at crisps and convenience foods should not be encouraged, as this spoils the appetite for the wholesome food which is so necessary at this stage of development.

Food for the toddler may be taken from the family pot, provided that it is not too highly seasoned. To encourage wholesome eating, it should vary in taste and in texture and should of course, be balanced. Food that encourages chewing is good not only for digestion, but for strengthening the jaws. The food can be cut into bite-sized bits as the toddler likes to use his hands when feeding himself. This will make feeding time much longer, and sometimes messier, but it is well worth the time spent in order to help in the child's development of independence. The toddler sitting up in a high chair at table soon begins to feel part of the

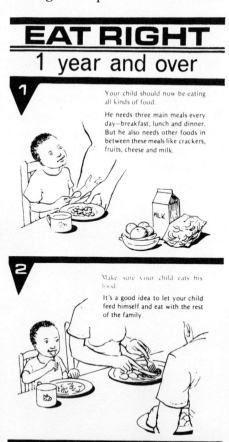

EAT RIGHT
1 year and over

1. Your child should now be eating all kinds of food.
   He needs three main meals every day—breakfast, lunch and dinner. But he also needs other foods in between these meals like crackers, fruits, cheese and milk.

2. Make sure your child eats his food.
   It's a good idea to let your child feed himself and eat with the rest of the family.

family, and this is also an opportunity for helping his social development.

Refusing food

Toddlers seem to thrive on three or four good meals each day, served at the same times. They should not be encouraged to eat snacks between meals. Mealtimes should not be hurried and the child should be taught to chew food slowly and thoroughly. After meals, the child should rest; this helps the digestion of the food. From time to time, a child may lose his appetite; this may be due to a cold or other illness coming on, or emotional upsets such as: a parent going away; the family moving house; or a death in the family. When the child feels better, or when the home situation returns to normal, the appetite usually returns.

A dislike for a particular food may develop after someone else in the family has expressed a dislike for it, or the food may be presented in an unattractive manner, which puts the child off, as in the case of the boy who explained to his parents that he could only eat aubergine if he closed his eyes; some grated cheese and breadcrumbs sprinkled on top and

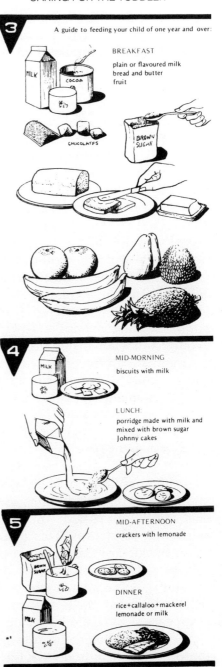

A guide to feeding your child of one year and over:

BREAKFAST
plain or flavoured milk
bread and butter
fruit

MID-MORNING
biscuits with milk

LUNCH
porridge made with milk and mixed with brown sugar
Johnny cakes

MID-AFTERNOON
crackers with lemonade

DINNER
rice + callaloo + mackerel
lemonade or milk

From 'Eat Right, 1 year and over', Ministry of Health, Kingston, Jamaica browned in the oven made all the difference to the appearance of the vegetable and he no longer had to close his eyes to eat it.

The child should not be forced to eat food which he dislikes, but encouraged to try it, small portions at a time. Example is also a good method to persuade children that a particular food is tasty; if the person feeding the child eats the same food and looks as if they are enjoying it, he might be tempted to try it.

When parents or those caring for the young child are worried that there is a feeding problem, it is advisable to have the child thoroughly examined by the doctor. If nothing is wrong physically, no fuss should be made if food is refused. Meals should be attractively served in the child's own brightly coloured containers, and in small portions. When a sufficiently long time has passed, and the child insists that he does not want any more of the food, it is best if it is removed without comment. Sometimes the toddler is distracted at mealtime by too much activity, such as other children and adults coming and going, or the television or loud music on the radio or stereo. It may be necessary to sit alone with him. If the child is made to feel that the adults are being granted a favour if and when meals are eaten, soon refusing food will be used as a method of attracting the parents' attention or getting his own way. A child will not usually starve himself and, though the amount eaten may appear small to the adult, it is usually satisfying.

THUMB SUCKING

One childhood habit which causes some parents to be unkind to the child is thumb sucking. In order to discourage the habit the thumb is tied, put in splints or rubbed with pepper or bad-tasting substances. This should *not* be done.

Sucking of the thumb begins in infancy. The baby satisfies his natural desire to suck and may put the thumb or other fingers in his mouth. Some infants who are left hungry for a long time may suck the thumb or the tongue or the bedclothes. Usually, this habit disappears as the child grows up.

In the toddler, the sucking may be satisfying the need for comfort. Some children suck the thumb before going to sleep, or if they have hurt themselves, are sad for any reason, feeling tired, or bored with no suitable activity and no toys with which to play.

Usually the average toddler who is secure in the family, and kept stimulated during the daytime gives up thumb sucking before being ready for nursery school or very soon after starting school. Some may return to the habit if illness strikes, or if there is a new baby in the family and attention is sought.

The persistent thumb sucker can be encouraged to give up the habit, but punishing and bribing and teasing only serve to reinforce it.

TEMPER TANTRUMS

From the earliest days of the baby's life, he is able to show anger. Although some babies are good-tempered, most of them will scream and kick if they are not fed when hungry, or if feeding is interrupted. When older, if he is restrained from trying to perform some action or touching some object, there may be screams, holding the breath or banging the head in a fit of rage.

The toddler, who as yet has very little self-control, may get into a temper and show this by biting or kicking. Adults should remain calm to help to quieten the child. Getting into a temper and shouting and slapping usually makes the situation worse.

If the child is in danger of hurting himself, for example by head-banging, he should be held firmly but gently for a few moments; this seems to be more comforting and reassuring than speaking.

Temper tantrums tend to occur in families where the child is spoken to negatively most of the time, and where no alternatives are given, or where no one listens to him.

Situations which provoke anger should be avoided. For example, when it is feeding time, mother or caretaker should devote time to this and not suddenly stop in order to answer the telephone at length; the caller may be asked to ring later.

It must also be remembered that children imitate. If the adults around are often angry, stamping and shouting, then the young child will imitate this behaviour.

TOILET TRAINING

Some parents are very anxious about having the children toilet trained at an early age, and long for the time when they are dry and use their potties.

The time at which toilet training begins varies considerably from country to country. In most western countries, it does not begin until well into the second year, while in other countries it may begin much earlier, with the baby being held over the pot at regular intervals from a very early age.

The baby has no control over muscles which control the bladder, so that urine is passed without any awareness that this is being done. There is also no control over bowel motions. Gradually, careful observation will show that the child is becoming aware of the discomfort caused by the need for a bowel movement. The child makes certain noises or certain squirming movements, and at times like these he may be held out on the potty.

It would seem most useful to put the child on the pot when he is able to sit on it on his own, and to do this at regular intervals, for example, after awakening, after a meal and before being put to bed.

Whenever training starts, accidents will always happen, and it is most important that the parents do not punish the child, but simply encourage him. Punishment will make the training a point of contention, and it will inevitably then take longer.

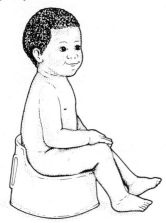

Sitting comfortably

Sometimes a toddler who has been trained to use the potty may begin to regress and wet or soil clothes or the floor. This is usually due to a change in the child's circumstances: there may be a new baby in the family who is attracting mother's attention; a change of staff in the day nursery; or some other emotional upset. Some parents try returning to nappies for a short time, and this may work if the child dislikes being treated as a baby. It is important that the child is gently treated at this time, and reassured of the parents' love, even though this may be time-consuming.

MASTURBATION

During the early months of their development, babies usually become interested in their bodies. They play with their fingers and toes, and may discover that when they touch their genitals a pleasant sensation is experienced. They may continue to do this, much to the annoyance and shame of the parents, who do not realise that most children do this at some stage. The normal healthy child will drop the habit as he grows older, if his needs for love and comfort are being met, and there are enough play materials and interesting activities to suit his stage of development.

If this habit persists up to the time the child is ready for nursery school, it is advisable to discuss it with the teacher who, with an understanding of human growth and development will not punish or shame the child, but provide a variety of activities, and perhaps give him extra jobs such as sharing out the crayons and collecting them, so that there will not be too much extra time spent alone and unoccupied.

Threatening to 'beat' the child or calling him 'bad' will only serve to create more anxiety and more need for comfort, so the habit will persist.

ANSWERING CHILDREN'S QUESTIONS

If the toddler is of normal intelligence, and has been properly nourished and feels loved and secure, he will have an interest in his surroundings and by the age of three will begin to ask questions. Some parents are very pleased about this, because they realise that the child is developing intellectually. Others may think the child is difficult and asks too many questions, some of which they are unable to answer such as: 'What is the moon made of?'

The toddler's first questions are about the things he sees and he wants to know 'What is that?' If the mother does not know, the child should not be given an untrue reply. The child might be told that the answer is not known but, 'We will ask someone who knows.' If the parent has been in the habit of answering the questions the child will accept this reply and wait until the answer is found out.

When the child discovers the question 'Why?' the adult finds difficulty keeping up with all the questions beginning with this. Sometimes the questions may seek information, but they may also be an attempt to avoid doing something. Sometimes the child who seeks attention may carry on asking 'Why?' even when he is given an answer. When this happens he can be reminded that the answer has already been given, and asked to repeat the answer. Most times he is able to do this accurately.

Answers should be in simple, straightforward language with not too much information given at a time, nor should adults tell untruths in answer to the child's questions. When a child discovers that parents have lied, this can very easily undermine trust and respect. It is very important to be patient and respond readily to the child as this helps his intellectual development.

USE OF OBSCENE LANGUAGE

Sometimes toddlers begin to use obscene words in the course of their play, or in reply to adults' questions which may interrupt their activity. Adults are very often shocked at the accuracy with which the child uses the word or phrase.

When the parents are amused and the child sees this, the word is repeated more often. Very often, if the word is ignored as if it was not heard, the child quickly stops using it. If the child repeats the word in an attempt to get some reaction from adults, he may be told that everybody is tired of hearing that word, and asked to use some of the other words which he knows.

If the child is angry and uses obscene words, he may be imitating an adult in or out of the house who has reacted this way. His correct use of the word or expression shows that he is developing mentally, and therefore needs examples of other ways of self-expression.

JEALOUSY

Jealousy is a very strong emotion which the young child shows after the birth of a new baby in the family. Preparation can reduce jealousy. The child can be encouraged to feel the baby move in the womb, or he can be involved in sorting out the baby's clothes, or any activity that makes him feel useful.

Many mothers recall the times when the toddler has tried pulling the baby off the bed or, beginning to kiss the baby, turns to biting it. These are ways in which the child shows resentment and unhappiness. Punishing the child by beating will only reinforce the feelings that he is no longer loved and the mother prefers the baby.

With care and planning a lot of jealousy is easily avoided. For example, a situation that needs careful handling is when mother comes home from hospital with the new baby. One way is for the child to be out – perhaps buying the new baby a present – when mother arrives home with the baby in her arms. By the time the child returns the mother is free to make a fuss over him before showing the new baby. If the child is at home, another way is for father to carry the new baby so that mother has her arms free to greet her older child. The important thing is never to exclude the older child or make too big a fuss over the new baby.

In the day-to-day care, the toddler can assist in handing things such as the powder to the mother, and in this way he begins to feel included in the care of the baby. Sometimes he may ask permission to hold the baby. This can be allowed for a few minutes, making sure that he is sitting well back in a big chair and an adult is near-by.

At times the toddler behaves like the baby, wetting or soiling clothes during the day and wetting the bed at night. He may refuse to drink from a cup and insist on a bottle, cry and be generally fretful and may refuse to go to nursery school. Even though this behaviour will be very annoying and cause extra work for the mother, it is best if he is allowed to behave like a baby for a little while, and a little extra attention given. This is the time that father can be very helpful to the toddler, playing with him and taking him out. Gradually the behaviour will return to normal.

Understanding of the toddler's feelings, of his age and stage of development, and therefore of his needs, will help the adults in the family to cope with this trying time. Patience is very much needed to demonstrate to the child that he is also loved. He should not be sent away to grandmother or anyone else for any length of time because this will only serve to reinforce the feeling that he is being pushed out by the baby. If this period of adjusting to sharing love and affection with a younger brother or sister is not properly handled, it may continue into later life.

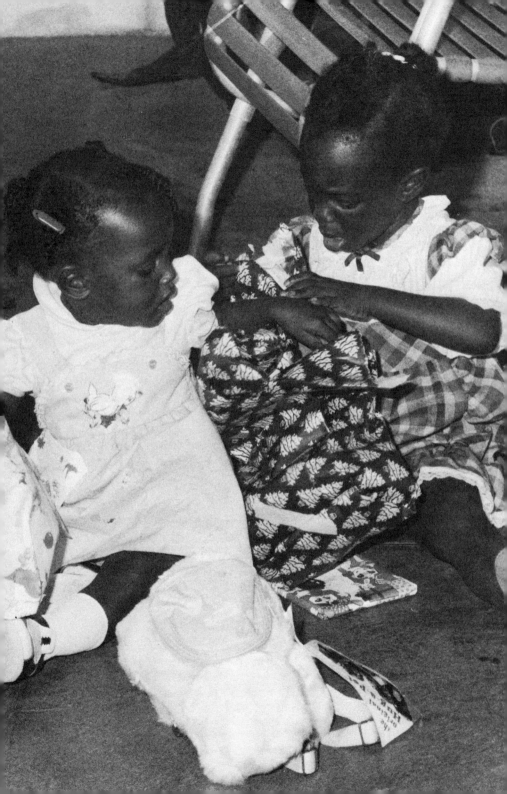

11 The value of play

Play may be described as a physical or mental activity which gives the individual pleasure and a feeling of accomplishment.

Children pass through many stages of growth and development before they arrive at maturity, and at every stage play aids their growth. Movement is important for the development of bones and muscles, and from the first attempts to hold the finger of an adult the child is trying to engage in exercise. During the daily routine opportunities should be given for the child to kick her legs without the restriction of clothing.

In her play certain skills will be learnt:

- **Body skills**: that is, the moving of arms and legs, and, later, walking, running, climbing, balancing.
- **Language skills**: talking, asking and answering questions.
- **Social skills**: eating, dressing, acceptance of social standards, such as co-operating with others.

Vision and fine movements will also develop as will the co-ordination of eye and hand movements when drawing, writing, sewing, hammering, and so on.

THE BABY AND PLAY

When the baby is about three months old, as she lies in her cot she will be observed kicking her legs, moving her arms and sometimes playing with her fingers. Later, sitting up in her cot or high chair, she will throw toys out and enjoy having them picked up and returned. Squeals of delight will accompany the return of the toy, and if the adult is not careful the 'game' can go on indefinitely. Later still, she will begin to play at peeping behind fingers and will clap hands and wave goodbye. At this stage the baby loves to play with an adult, and this gives father and other relatives the opportunity to become involved with the child. Care must be taken nevertheless not to over-stimulate the child immediately before bedtime.

A playpen

A playpen is a useful piece of furniture when a new baby joins the family, as, from about the age of four months, it affords protection for the baby when mother or caretaker is busy with household chores. At this stage of development the baby is able to reach for and hold objects, is taking an interest in people and things and needs a change from the cot or pram.

The size and shape of the playpen will depend on the space available in the home. The safe pen is one which is well-constructed with smooth wood that does not splinter. There should be no protruding nails or hinges and, if painted, the paint should be non-toxic. The bars should not be wide enough for the baby's head to go through, and there should be enough space in the pen for the baby to roll and kick with her toys around. The bars and the sides of the pen provide support for the child to pull herself up as she grows. Some families who are unable to purchase or make a pen improvise with boxes or backs of chairs. These too need to be safe.

Some children, as they begin to crawl and move around, object to being put into the confined space for any length of time. Parents should be tolerant of this and not insist on keeping the child there if she cries persistently and clearly shows a desire to get out. Often it is a good idea to let her crawl around the floor for a change, and she might not object to being put back in with a favourite toy until it is time for feed or bath.

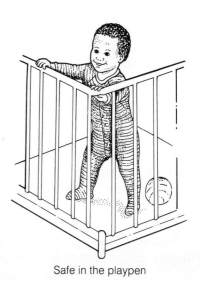

Safe in the playpen

It is usually a good idea to get the child used to being in the playpen before she can crawl freely around the floor, as otherwise she will object to the sudden restriction. Never put her in the playpen to punish her or she will begin to associate the pen with unhappy feelings.

TYPES OF PLAY

Babies and young children will not play *with* each other, but *alongside* one another, only showing interest in the other child when they want that child's toy.

There are various types of play:

- **Active play**: which helps the child to develop physically and provides the opportunity to use up energy.
- **Imaginative play**: children love to pretend and to dress up. In their games of make-believe they act out much that they observe in daily life. The adults around soon get a very clear idea of how they behave by watching the children at play. Young children also act out some of their fears or anxieties. For example, after having an injection children may be observed giving injections to their dolls or to each other. They may also get rid of some of their angry feelings when they play at the parent scolding the child.
- **Creative play**: children very often express ideas in the things they make before they are able to describe them with words.
- **Explorative play**: from the time the baby is able to crawl, search and exploration begin. This way she learns about the world around her.
- **Fun play**: for sheer relaxation and enjoyment.
- **Rough play**: some babies seem to enjoy rough play which may include being tossed up and down, whilst others do not; if the child does not enjoy it, the adult should not persist.

TOYS

Just as adults need tools with which to work, children need tools with which to play; the tools are toys and play materials. Toys and play materials need not be expensive, and may be provided from lots of household items usually thrown away:

- boxes and cartons of all sizes
- thread spools
- the middle of toilet rolls
- paper bags
- old newspapers
- old socks for puppets
- strips of various coloured paper attached to an old clothes hanger for an attractive mobile
- plastic bottles with some beans for a musical instrument

Care of course should be taken against giving children glass bottles which may be easily broken, or tins with rough edges. Bear the following points in mind when choosing toys:

1. The toys must be suitable for the age and stage of the child's development.
2. They must be safe; no rough edges. If painted, the paint must be non-toxic. The material must not be easily broken.
3. They must be well-made and able to stand up to rough handling.
4. The toys must be made of material which can be easily cleaned.
5. The toys should be attractive in appearance and should appeal to the child.
6. Some of the toys must be capable of being used in different ways, e.g. blocks which can be used to build a house or train.
7. Toys for the young child should be free of buttons or other small objects which may be swallowed.

Knowing how the child develops helps the adults in selecting suitable toys. It has been stated repeatedly that children develop at different rates, but there is a pattern to the development.

Keen observation is necessary so that the child may not be given toys or material too difficult to be handled. This causes frustration which may lead to destruction. On the other hand, if the material is too simple, this may cause boredom and disinterest.

It is important to look at the order of development and not take the child's age into account only. The following gives a rough guide to the type of toys suitable for different ages:

0–6 months	Contact with an adult is the most important thing. The baby loves the human voice and to see a face. Very few toys are needed: a mobile hung over the cot; rubber toys; a rattle.
6–12 months 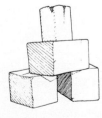	The child is still interested in playing with an adult. Most things are put into the mouth. It is important the toys are too big to be swallowed. Suitable toys: washable toys such as rubber animals; wooden reels; anything that can rattle; boxes or old saucepans which can be filled and emptied; a sealed tin or plastic bottle with seeds or stones; brightly-coloured, medium-sized balls; big wooden beads on a string; floating toy for the bath; cloth or board books.

THE VALUE OF PLAY

1–2 years

This is a year of rapid development. The child needs space to move. The adult is still needed, for example to read to her. The following will always be useful: push-and-pull toys; building blocks; rubber balls; boxes large enough for climbing in and out; rubber dolls; pail and spade; sandbox; wooden hammer and pegs; low swings; a small table and chair; a small slide.

2–3 years

The child at this stage needs ample opportunities for physical activities such as running, climbing, swinging etc. She will enjoy being read to more and more, and talking with adults. The following toys will be used: imitation household toys, e.g. ironing boards, pots and pans, telephone; cars, trucks and fire engines; musical instruments; modelling clay or play dough; paper and finger paint; wheelbarrow; tricycle; picture books; or outdoors: climbing frames; swings and slides; suspended tyres; barrels to climb through; wading pools.

3–4 years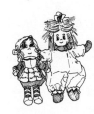

The child begins to enjoy playing with other children of her own age. She is more interested in looking at picture books and listening to stories, painting and drawing. Large sheets of paper, large brushes, chalk blocks, balls of various sizes, toys on wheels, dolls' clothes and furniture, clothes for dressing up and plasticine are all invaluable. She enjoys action songs and finger plays.

4–5 years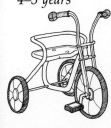

The child is beginning to be ready to leave the safety of home for school. She is able to play more imaginatively on her own and able to play and share toys with other children such as a bat and ball, toy scissors and paper, a child-sized playhouse, see-saw, tricycle, doctor's and nurse's kits, workmen's tools.

THE EARLY YEARS

Quantity of toys

Children sometimes are given so many toys that they become confused. They may select a few favourite ones and ignore the others, or they play with an article of no value and leave the expensive toys untouched. A child will play with the article which meets her needs at a particular stage of development. The household objects which stretch the imagination are always useful. A chair could become a boat, or a starship. A new toy for special occasions such as illness or disappointment – having to stay in on a rainy day – very often helps to make the child less unhappy.

If relatives and friends give too many toys on birthdays and at Christmas, some may be put away and brought out at a later date.

Putting toys away

'A place for everything and everything in its place' is a good and useful motto in the home. A large box put in a corner of the room where the very young child can see the toys being put away helps to give her the idea at an early age that toys must not be left scattered around. The toddler needs to be reminded by the adults in the family to put the toys in the box. Clearing away can also be a source of fun. Young children love to see 'who can finish first'.

Sometimes when playing with paper, bits may be left on the floor; most children enjoy clearing up whilst adults sing the following rhyme, which children soon learn and join in:

Lots of toys, lots of toys

or:

Bits of paper, bits of paper,
Lying on the floor, lying on the floor,
Make the place untidy, make the place untidy,
Pick them up, pick them up.

Parents who train the young child in habits of tidying will be well rewarded when she grows older and does not leave belongings scattered around the house.

SUPERVISION OF PLAY

In the home where children are wanted, parents are able to build a satisfying relationship with them in the very earliest stages. These parents usually find it easy to play with their children.

When a young child invites an adult to play, it is much better if the child is allowed to take the lead. It can be very surprising how well she is able to give instructions for the games, especially those of make-believe.

It is necessary that some of the child's activities must be supervised to ensure safety, but adults must be careful not to express too many 'don'ts'. This tends to make the child timid and nervous about experimenting. If the child tries to perform acts unsuitable to her strength or beyond her control, it should be suggested that the activity may be done when she is bigger and stronger; most children understand and will stop.

CLOTHES FOR PLAY

Because toddlers are very busy little people, they must be dressed in comfortable clothes and those suitable for play activities. It is pointless putting young children in expensive clothes and telling them not to dirty them. Toddlers' clothes should be of durable material which can be easily washed. Attention should be paid to the fitting of their underwear – tight elastic bands can be very uncomfortable.

THE IMAGINARY PLAYMATE

Make-believe play is a normal activity through which the child expresses his imagination. This begins about the age of two years in the average child, who may pretend to eat the fruits and vegetables out of picture books and to share these with her favourite adults. She may pretend to be a train, a bus, an aeroplane, the postman who delivers letters, or an animal which is going to eat everybody up.

About this time, or a year later, many children begin to invent a playmate who may be of the same sex and is there at mealtimes and at bedtimes. Sometimes some of the toys with which the playmate may play are put aside. Sometimes the imaginary playmate may be the one who does all the wrong things, who wets the bed, or spills the juice or refuses to put away the toys.

Some parents who are superstitious become very worried about the child talking about someone else who is not really there, and feel that the child is playing with 'spirits'. They may take the child to the priest or to someone who has the reputation for removing spirits. This is totally unnecessary. In time, when the child gets a little older she stops this imaginary play.

Parents should accept the 'playmate' and talk about him or her with the child. They will soon realise that the child is aware that it is make-believe. If however the child continues throughout all of her play to prefer her imaginary playmate to children of her own age, it may be that there is some problem which is giving her difficulty in adjusting to the real world. Parents should consider whether they have been giving enough attention to the child and communicating or playing when they are invited to do so (especially if the child is an only child). If they are in any doubt, they may seek advice from the nursery teacher, social worker or a doctor.

OUTDOOR PLAY

Outings to parks and savannahs and to the beaches provide an opportunity for the child to play in wide open spaces. Usually in the playparks there is equipment which serves to test muscular development – swings, climbing frames, slides, sandpits, see-saws and merry-go-rounds.

Care must be taken that the playing areas are safe, free from broken bottles, old tins, pieces of old wood with rusty nails, and holes. The play equipment should be firmly placed in the ground and wooden seats should be free from splinters. The ropes and chains of swings and bolts of climbing frames and see-saws should be periodically checked.

When children are taken to these play areas, the adults should check on all of these things and keep a watchful eye during the playtime. Too often adults let the children free whilst they sit and talk with one another, and without warning an accident occurs due to lack of supervision.

Parents may not be able to afford some of the bigger pieces of play equipment found in the grounds of a good nursery school or a public park, but it may be possible to hang a swing or used car tyre on a tree in the garden. The same standards of safety should be maintained.

SWIMMING

Most young children love the water and are capable of learning to swim at an early age. Some parents are able to afford to have them taught in swimming pools, but in the Caribbean islands the vast majority will more likely take the child to the river or the sea.

To the toddler the large expanse of water, with the waves breaking on the shore can be frightening. She may refuse to go in the water, even in the strong arms of her father. On no account should force be used or the child called silly or a coward. An adult or older child may sit with her at the water's edge where she can get her feet wet, and make sand castles or dig with her spade and bucket. The more often the toddler is taken to the beach, the more familiar the sea becomes, and, as she notices the enjoyment of others and their safe return to the shore, she may venture in with a trusted adult. Rough seas with big waves should be avoided, and at all times the child should wear water-wings or arm-bands as a safety measure.

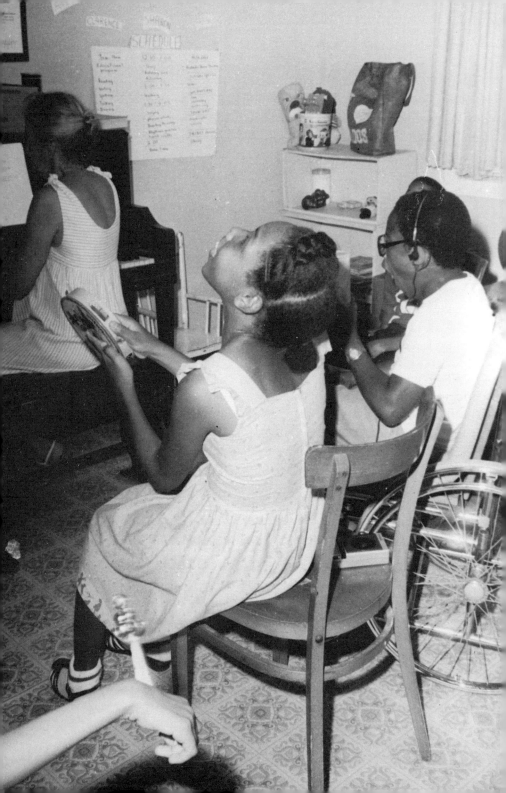

12 The handicapped child

A child who has a recognisable persistent physical or mental defect which prevents normal development and prevents participation in the activities important to growing children, is considered to be handicapped. Included are those disabled by loss of sight, hearing, by crippling deformity, by extensive damage to the heart or central nervous system, as well as those with mental retardation.

Initially the parents may be shocked and disappointed or they may be angry and ask 'Why me?'. They may both feel guilty or one may blame the other; but the commonest reaction is one of grief, especially if the child is the first, to which they were eagerly looking forward.

One fact needs to be borne in mind: a handicapped child may be born into any family, rich or poor, educated or uneducated, healthy or diseased.

CAUSES OF HANDICAP

Handicaps are either **congenital**, that is, existing at birth, or acquired after birth.

Congenital abnormalities

The following lists some of the reasons for congenital abnormality:

1 The nervous system and heart do not develop properly in the womb
2 Infections, such as rubella (German measles) contracted by the mother during the first 12 weeks of pregnancy
3 Drugs, such as thalidomide, or X-rays to the abdomen during the first 12 weeks
4 Down's syndrome, formerly known as mongolism, caused by the presence of an extra chromosome at conception
5 There is a malformation of the baby's spine, resulting in the condition known as **spina bifida**

Acquired abnormalities

These are caused by damage to various organs from birth onwards and may arise from lack of oxygen (especially during a long and difficult labour), infection or poisoning.

EARLY DIAGNOSIS AND TREATMENT

In countries where health visitors visit mother and baby regularly after delivery, the chances of early detection of a handicap are increased. The parents then obtain information about the condition and referrals to the specialist for confirmation of diagnosis and treatment as soon as possible. Some parents find it very difficult to accept the diagnosis of mental retardation and, if they are able to afford the fees, they consult doctor after doctor in the hope that some cure can be found. In these instances the family can be helped by the family doctor, social worker, nurse or relatives to accept the problem and to find the best way of helping the child.

THE NEEDS OF THE HANDICAPPED CHILD

The handicapped child has all the needs of the normal child. He needs love, even though at times he may not be able to return this, companionship and proper physical care. There are also specific needs to be met according to the type of handicap. For example, the blind child needs to learn through touch and sound and smell, so therefore the adults in the family should help to provide the experiences to meet these needs.

There are times when the child may be cared for at home, but, if the handicap is severe, then he may be cared for in an institution where there are people trained and qualified to meet his needs and help him to develop whatever skills are possible.

Special care

In some countries there are special schools for the physically handicapped and transport is provided to assist parents in getting their children to attend. The staff are specially trained and classes are smaller, allowing the children to develop at their individual rates.

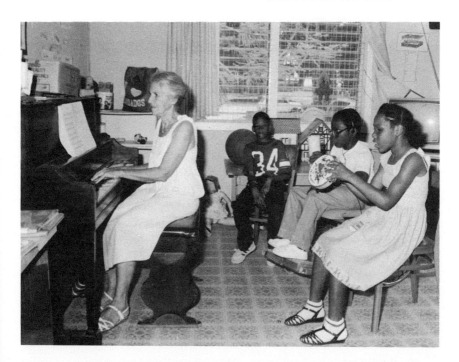

Handicapping conditions which frequently cause children to be cared for in institutions are Down's syndrome where the child is cared for in a home for the mentally retarded and spina bifida where he is cared for in a home for the physically handicapped. They may be looked after in these institutions because they are members of a large family where space is limited or mother needs to work, or the doctor advises that the child would be better cared for away from home.

Some institutions caring for the handicapped child arrange classes for parents in order to help them understand the nature of the handicap and also how they may cope at home during the holidays with the child. It is essential that parents maintain contact with children in institutions.

Unfortunately, in the rural and poorer areas these facilities are not usually available. Some children may be placed in residential homes but the waiting lists are usually long and many remain at home without the benefit of proper care and the development of their potential.

CARE OF A CHILD WITH DOWN'S SYNDROME

This form of handicap was formerly called mongolism because the deep folds in the skin around the slanted eyes gave the appearance of people of Mongolian origin. The name was misleading as the condition has nothing to do with this country. Finally the name was changed and called after the doctor who discovered its cause.

The baby is very quiet and placid, seldom crying for attention and some mothers may mistakenly think that he is 'a good baby'. The physical development is much slower than that of the normal child and colds and chest complaints are more frequent. Feeding takes an extra long time as coaxing is needed to interest him in taking the food. With extra stimulation the child will pass the various milestones and become capable of doing routine activities. Many Down's syndrome children excel in an appreciation of rhythm and music.

Most of these children are happy, loving and affectionate and attract loving attention from parents, brothers and sisters and indeed from all who come in contact with them, but care needs to be taken that overprotection does not prevent them from being trained to their full potential.

Some hospitals or voluntary organisations for work with the mentally retarded organise group sessions for mothers of Down's syndrome children where the feelings about having a retarded child are discussed and where professionals can help and advise on suitable activities for the stimulation of the individual child.

The condition seems more likely to occur with the first child of older parents or after several normal healthy children. But it is also possible for younger mothers to have a baby with the condition.

OTHER CHILDREN IN THE FAMILY

When there are other children in the family, sometimes they may become jealous of the extra attention that is given to the handicapped child, and so parents should include them as much as possible in helping to care for their brother or sister and explain why the attention is necessary. The children will model their reactions to the retarded child on their parents. If the parents are not ashamed or embarrassed, the other children will, in most instances, love and protect the child and so help him to be accepted in the family.

Generally there is not adequate provision for the care of handicapped children in the community, and families need to do the best they can with caring for their children. If they are able to accept the child with his handicap, and learn as much as they can about the condition, and if all of the family members are co-operative and give help and support, the life of the handicapped child can be made very happy.

Sometimes having such a child in the family helps to bring out qualities of love, patience and understanding and tolerance of human beings which help the individual members in their own self-development and their dealing with people in the wider community.

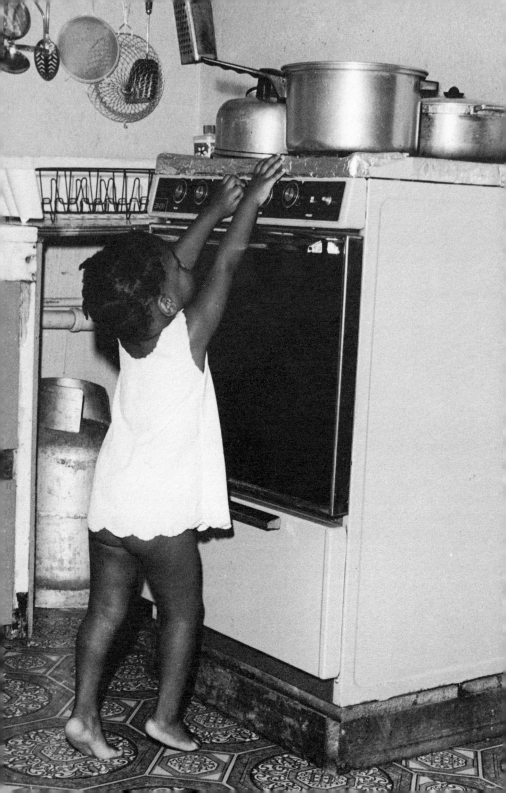

13 Illness and accidents

Parents or anyone caring for the baby or toddler should consult the health visitor, clinic nurse or doctor if they suspect the child is ill. On no account should they ask a chemist to give a medicine for any ailment. This should always be prescribed by a doctor.

Most children during infancy and early childhood suffer from one or other of the common infectious diseases. It is usually when toddlers start to attend nursery school that infections are passed from one to the other. After recovering from some of these infections such as chicken pox, a resistance, known as **immunity**, to the illness is built up.

WHEN IS A DOCTOR NEEDED?

A normally healthy child will recover from most slight infections without medical help. Sometimes there may be a slightly raised temperature; this is the body's defence against infection.

The child will most likely be better after a good night's sleep, but if the raised temperature persists and there is also a runny nose and a slight cough, probably these are signs of the beginning of the common cold.

The parent or adult caring for the baby or toddler from day to day will be the one who is best able to judge when it is necessary to call the doctor or to take the child to be examined.

In the young baby, if some of the following occur a doctor should be contacted immediately:

- No interest in feeds
- Unaccustomed quietness and weak crying
- Convulsions
- Diarrhoea and vomiting
- Difficulty in breathing: panting or choking
- Bleeding of any kind
- A blow on the head
- Burns or scalds

With the toddler, if she has a high temperature accompanied by any of the following the doctor should be contacted:

- A rash
- Severe pain in the head, neck, ears causing persistent crying
- Extreme paleness
- Strange behaviour such as agitation and inability to keep still, or listlessness and staring

When the doctor is contacted, the symptoms should be clearly stated, giving the exact times when they began. If there is any suspicion that the child may have swallowed some foreign substance such as pills meant for someone else in the family, or liquid from an unlabelled bottle, the containers or bottles should be taken along to the doctor.

CARING FOR THE SICK CHILD

When a baby is ill, the adults around become very distressed because of her inability to tell where the pain is located, or how she feels.

The doctor's instructions should be very carefully followed. It may be that there is need to take the baby's temperature to report to the doctor, so that a check is kept on the baby's progress. Most babies do not fuss when their temperatures are taken if the adult is gentle and unexcited. The clinic nurse will demonstrate how this is done during antenatal classes. If in any doubt, however, when the actual necessity for taking the temperature arises, help should be sought from the health visitor.

Time should be spent giving the baby the extra cuddling which will be of comfort. Instead of putting on lots of clothes and covering the child up, light, cool coverings should be used. Cool or tepid sponging will help to lower the fever.

Infectious illnesses deprive the body of water – this is known as **dehydration** – so the child should be given plenty to drink. If there is vomiting, sips of glucose and water seem to help. Infections also increase the body's need for vitamin C. This vitamin is found in citrus and other fruits, so the child can be given juices of locally-grown fruit, and there is no need to buy expensive imported juices.

ILLNESS AND ACCIDENTS

If the doctor prescribes antibiotics, either in liquid form or in tablets, the directions must be closely followed. If there is any adverse reaction, this should be reported to the doctor immediately. Even when the child gets better in the middle of the course of tablets, the entire course should be taken. The antibiotics should not be saved up for another illness, and they should not be given to any other member of the family.

If the toddler has to be kept in bed, a favourite toy may help in amusing her. Mobiles can be hung over the bed and changed from time to time to prevent boredom. The adults in the family may read or tell stories, and look at picture books together with the child. She may be very fretful and demanding but, if provided with a variety of toys and play material she should amuse herself for part of the day.

When the child begins to feel better and gets out of bed, care must be taken that she does not get overtired.

IMMUNISATION

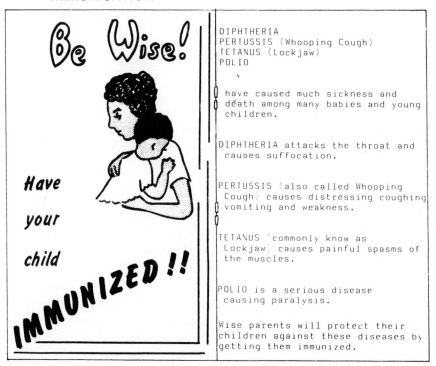

From 'Be wise', Bureau of Health Education, Kingston, Jamaica

Today, thanks to modern medicine, the young child is protected against many infectious diseases through **immunisation**. Immunisation means that a protective substance is given which helps the body to resist or fight against the germs which cause the disease. The protection may last for a long time after one injection, or there may be need for booster doses of medicine. For polio, the vaccine is given by mouth.

Immunisation is free and easily obtainable through child welfare clinics and health offices or in offices of private doctors.

The times when immunisation is started against the various diseases can be checked during antenatal classes, and later with doctor or clinic nurse. All instructions should be carefully followed and the baby taken for booster doses when advised.

In some countries the child will not be admitted to day nurseries, nursery or infant schools unless a fully completed Immunisation Card is presented as evidence that the child has been immunised. Children are immunised against the following in most countries:

- Whooping cough
- Measles
- Diphtheria
- Tetanus
- Polio myelitis

COMMON INFECTIONS

Infection of the eye

Because the importance of good healthy eyes is recognised by everyone interested in the care of the young child, special attention is paid to them from the time of birth. The doctor examines them carefully and makes sure there is no infection. When the baby is bathed, each eye should be cleaned with its own piece of cotton wool squeezed out of cooled boiled water, but a common problem among babies is the blocking of a tear duct (which is a little canal that drains tear fluid from the eye to the nose). The eye waters more profusely as a result of the blocking. The eyelids become infected and a whitish discharge forms along the edges and sometimes forms a crust which sticks the lids down. The eye should be cleaned with sterile cotton wool moistened with tepid boiled water.

Conjunctivitis

If the toddler is observed to be constantly rubbing the eyes it may be that she is suffering from an eye infection known as **conjunctivitis**. There are several forms of this disease and some of the symptoms are pink or red eyeballs, swelling and pain in the eye, a dislike of light and a discharge of pus. Parents should not waste time by trying home remedies. Water that has been boiled and cooled can be used to wash the eyelids, and the child should be taken to the doctor at the very earliest opportunity.

Some forms of eye infections can be contagious, and the child should have her own wash cloth, and tissues used to wipe the eyes should be disposed of down the lavatory or burnt.

The child's hands should be kept clean and she needs to be supervised in order to prevent excessive rubbing which further irritates the eyes.

Ear infections

It is surprising how many young children suffer with ear infections. A baby may suffer from earache which is usually indicated by her turning her head from side to side, and fretful crying. If there is a high temperature, the earache may be a sign of something more serious, and the doctor should be consulted immediately. Prompt treatment with the new drugs available can prevent a mild infection of the ear from developing into a serious one. Any discharge from the ear should be treated as serious, and the ear should be seen by a doctor.

Mastoiditis

This is inflammation of the **mastoid**, the bone just behind the ear. This usually occurs among children who have a chronic ear, nose or throat infection. Sometimes it may occur after an attack of measles. Fortunately, with antibiotic drugs, the condition is now not as frequent as it used to be, but parents need to be observant in noticing any ear infection and have this treated early. Besides the pain and discomfort which the child will suffer, there is the risk of poor development of language if she is not able to hear properly.

Colds

Before the baby has developed immunity to germs, colds may be a problem, and the nostrils may become blocked. Adults with colds should not hold or kiss the baby. Following several days with a cold, the baby may develop a hoarse crowing noise when breathing in. This is caused by an infection in the larynx and is called **croup**. It can be dangerous as breathing is impaired. The child should be seen by a doctor. While waiting for the doctor to relieve the breathing, the child should be kept warmly wrapped in the kitchen with the steam from a boiling kettle or pot filling the room. The clothes around the neck should be loose and the neck held straight.

Swollen glands

Sometimes the toddler suffers with swollen glands in the neck. This is a sign of infection and should be treated by a doctor.

Scabies

This condition is commonly called 'the itch'. It is caused by a parasite which bores its way into the skin and usually attacks between the fingers and toes, inside of the arms and between the legs and the buttocks. It is likely to occur if the child is not kept clean, but clean children may contract it if they come in contact with the skin of others suffering from it. Sometimes it may be contracted when attending nursery school. The nurse or doctor should be asked for advice on treatment.

CAUSE OF SOME INFECTIONS

Some mild infections occur when the toddler has a cold. The child may blow his nose too forcibly, holding both nostrils at the same time. This can force some of the infected mucus from the nose and throat into the ear. The child needs to be taught to blow the nose gently, one nostril at a time.

The ear is very delicate and probing the ear to remove wax with a hairpin or sharp object is dangerous; the ear may be scratched and can be easily infected. If there is hardened wax in the ear this should be removed only by a doctor.

ILLNESS AND ACCIDENTS

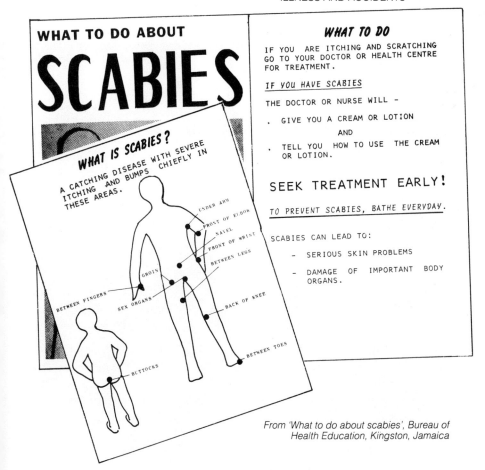

From 'What to do about scabies', Bureau of Health Education, Kingston, Jamaica

AVOIDANCE OF INFECTIONS

Although it is very difficult to avoid some infections, especially when the child is attending nursery school, maintaining a high standard of hygiene in the home will reduce the risks. If the child is suffering from any infectious diseases, any tissues used to wipe the nose should be flushed down the lavatory or burnt. The child's feeding utensils should be washed up separately from the rest of the family's.

Several diseases, such as **leptospirosis**, are contracted through eating food contaminated by rats, so floors should be thoroughly swept, and no food left uncovered.

THE EARLY YEARS

ILLNESS AND ACCIDENTS

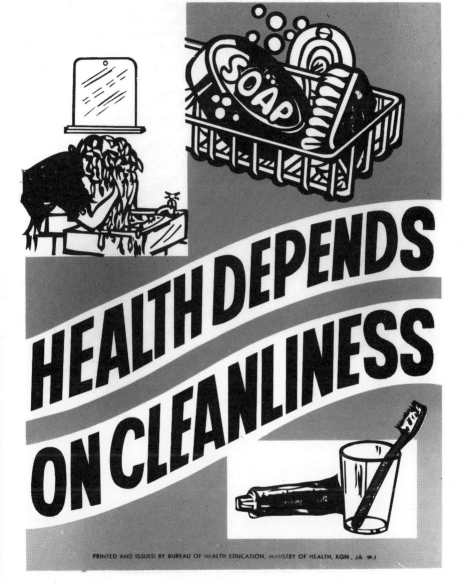

FIRST AID

No matter how careful those caring for children may be, accidents will sometimes happen, and a knowledge of first aid is essential. Anyone may take the courses in first aid run by the Red Cross or the St John Ambulance Brigade, and a first-aid book should be kept in the house for reference. First aid should be carried out gently and as quickly as possible, but medical treatment must always be sought when there is a serious accident, and a detailed account of the accident given to the doctor. Because the toddler is so very active, falls and bumps are frequent.

It is advisable to keep a first-aid box handy. This should include:

- a box of adhesive dressings (plasters) of various sizes
- a box of sterile gauze dressings of various sizes for cuts
- a packet of paper tissues to use as temporary sterile dressings
- two or three cotton bandages to put over the dressings to keep them in place
- two or three crepe bandages for sprains
- a triangular bandage or clean linen or cotton tea towel to use as a sling, or as a large dressing for a burn or scald
- small roll of cottonwool for padding
- blunt ended scissors
- safety pins and roll of adhesive tape for fastening dressings

Bruises

When the small blood vessels are injured this causes the skin to discolour and there may be swelling. The application of a cloth wrung out in cold water will usually relieve the pain. If bruises appear on the child's skin without her having knocked the spot or falling, this should be brought to the doctor's attention, in case it is a sign of a serious blood disease which starts in this way.

In some of the Caribbean islands, there are folk tales of the 'soucyant', believed to be an old woman able to shed her skin and fly about in a ball of light who sucks the blood of her victims. If a discoloured spot on the body is noticed on waking, those who are superstitious complain of the presence of a soucyant. The folk tale continues that the only way to rid the community of the soucyant is

ILLNESS AND ACCIDENTS

to find her skin, which she hides under a water barrel, and sprinkle it with salt. She will never be able to put this on again and will die.

Burns

Burns are caused by dry heat such as flame or electricity, and scalds by wet heat such as hot water and other liquids and chemicals. If the child's clothes are burning, she should be wrapped in a rug or coat and rolled on the floor or ground.

If the burn is very slight, cool with cold water – no oils or butter or grease should be applied. If the burn is severe, involving a large area of the body, the doctor must be consulted immediately. Any clothing sticking to the skin must *not* be removed. If conscious, the child should be given water to drink until the doctor arrives, or until the child arrives at the hospital and is treated for shock.

Shock

Any serious injury is usually followed by shock, the signs of which are:

- Paleness, faintness or weakness
- Dilated pupils and dull eyes
- Rapid but weak pulse
- Rapid, shallow and irregular breathing
- Vomiting
- Unconsciousness

The child should be kept warm so as to keep the normal body temperature at 37 °C. Rest and quiet are important. The child should be put to lie down with her feet slightly higher than her head. Small amounts of warm, sweetened fluid may be given but not if there is vomiting, an abdominal injury, or if the child is unconscious.

Insect bites

Mosquito and fly bites, especially on sensitive skin, can cause discomfort, and scratching may cause infection. The itching may be controlled by applying a paste of bicarbonate of soda or calamine lotion on a cold, wet cloth. Bee stings should be squeezed out and may be bathed with a weak solution of vinegar and water.

Toddlers should be warned against trying to catch bees and, in rural areas, against picking up pretty crawling things: these may turn out to be a deadly coral snake! The child should not be made afraid, but where the area is noted for insects and other animal life such as snakes, centipedes and scorpions, great care and supervision are necessary.

Bleeding

Most children are frightened by the sight of blood and need to be reassured and treated by a calm adult. Minor cuts should be cleaned with warm water, checked for splinters and covered with a small plaster dressing. In more severe cases of bleeding, pressure should be applied to stop the bleeding and the child taken to the doctor or nearest hospital.

Broken bones

A broken bone should not be moved. The injured limb may be bandaged to the body; an arm may be put in a sling until medical help is obtained.

Choking

This causes disruption of breathing and must be dealt with immediately. The child should be turned upside down and smacked sharply three or four times between the shoulder blades to dislodge the obstruction; gently holding the child afterwards will help to revive her and calm the fear caused by the difficulty in breathing.

Artificial respiration

This is used if the child stops breathing. Mouth-to-mouth respiration is more commonly used as it is so immediate. The head should be tilted backwards in order to open the air passage from mouth to the lungs, the nostrils squeezed together and then air blown through the child's mouth. This should be repeated at the adult's breathing rate until breathing is restored.

ILLNESS AND ACCIDENTS

Swallowing or pushing small objects in ears or nostrils

If a child swallows a small smooth object, a bulky feed of soft bread and milk or mashed potatoes should be given; the object is usually passed in the stool. The child should not be given a laxative.

If a safety pin or other sharp object is swallowed, the child should be taken to a doctor or hospital immediately.

When the baby begins to crawl and to pick up things, there is always the risk that a small object may be pushed into the ear or nose. The adult in the home should take the child to the hospital or doctor, and not try to remove it. The ear is very delicate and could be easily damaged by pushing into it with a hairpin, as is so frequently done by the inexperienced.

ACCIDENT PREVENTION

In most countries accidents are a major public health problem. In industrial countries machines at work and vehicles on the crowded streets take their toll on the lives of adults and children. In developing countries, accidents frequently occur when young children are left in the care of others who are not much older, or with the elderly and infirm who may be unable to supervise the active toddler. But whatever the country, in most instances, accidents in the home account for a high proportion of injuries to children.

Whenever there is severe damage done to the child or the accident proves fatal, there is a very depressing and devastating effect on the family who constantly feel guilty.

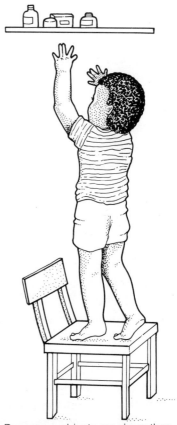
Dangerous objects are closer than mother imagines!

THE EARLY YEARS

Instilling safety habits in the young child is an excellent way of safeguarding their health. It must be remembered that, as the toddler and school child become less dependent on adults, there is more exposure to risks of injury, the dangers of which are compounded by the fact that they are not conscious of danger.

Between the ages one and three, when balance is still not mastered and walking is unsteady, the toddler may fall down steps, or face down in a pool of water. Some children have drowned by falling in a wash tub of water in the backyard, or in a swimming pool or in a nearby pond. Tubs and water barrels should be securely covered and a barrier placed in front of the door. This also prevents the four- or five-year-old from dashing out on to the street in front of an oncoming vehicle. Children should be trained to tell the adult what they would like to do and where they are going, despite the fact that they are spontaneous and act on the spur of the moment. Proper supervision is therefore necessary for, sad to say, many accidents take place in the presence of adults. Supervision does not mean over-protection and constant shouting of 'Don't do that!', but a surveying of the environment, alertness to possible dangers and setting limits for the child. Children in the company of each other are more daring and sometimes they enjoy showing off, so the adult should be at hand in case of reckless and dangerous behaviour.

Safety precautions

In the home

Most accidents are caused by carelessness in the home. Many could be prevented by taking the following precautions:

All medicines should be carefully stored out of reach and locked in a medicine chest. Tablets and capsules which are brightly coloured may be mistaken for sweets. The child may imitate the adult and swallow them if left lying around. The school child should be taught the danger codes on bottles and boxes and their meaning. For example, the skull and cross bones for poison.

Bleach, chemicals, kerosine, weed killer, should never be put in fruit drink or aerated drink bottles. These should be stored out of reach of the child in their proper containers.

Stools, chairs, low tables should be kept well away from open

ILLNESS AND ACCIDENTS

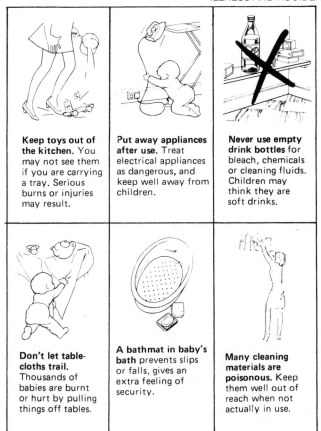

windows which may be high up off the ground and through which the child may climb.

Hanging table cloths should not be used when the child is crawling around; teapots and jugs of hot liquid can easily be pulled off by the child.

Toys must be cleared from the floor, especially in the kitchen or dining area where the adult may trip over them whilst carrying a pot of hot liquid, or a tray of dishes.

Electrical outlets should be covered, and the flex of the iron should not be left hanging from the ironing board.

Floors should not be highly polished, and the child should be taught to walk slowly and carefully on waxed floors. Rugs should be non-slip, and bare floors should be checked for splinters and small holes. The toddler could easily break a toe.

THE EARLY YEARS

Cupboard doors should be kept closed as the child may crawl in and fall asleep and could well be closed in. The shock of awakening in a dark confined space would be very frightening.

All sharp-edged tools, knives or scissors should be kept safely away. Where possible the toddler can be given play tools such as blunt-edged scissors as she will want to imitate adults.

Plastic bags should be kept out of reach as they can hamper breathing and cause suffocation if placed over the head.

Outdoors

Young children need to be warned of the following dangers:

Some plants can cause injury when grasped, for example, rose bushes, cacti, sisal.

Fruits should not be picked up from the ground and eaten without being washed, and more important without being shown to an adult, as some fruits and berries are poisonous.

Dogs and cats should not be teased and handled roughly, as they will bite or scratch. Unfamiliar dogs must not be touched. (This should be done without instilling fear of domestic animals.)

'Pretty' crawling things should not be played with. Some children have been known to pick up deadly coral snakes which are very attractive with colours of red, white and black.

Safety on the road

Many accidents occur on the road, either by children running out behind a ball or stepping off the curb or from behind parked vehicles into the way of oncoming traffic. The young child must be constantly warned against these dangers and wherever possible the following precautions taken:

Hold the toddler's hand when crossing a busy street, at the same time repeating the highway code of looking to both sides of the street and back again.

Teach the meaning of the colours of traffic lights and obey these strictly when in the presence of children.

Remind school children in rural areas to look out for tractors, and animal-drawn carts, especially during the cane or any other crop-harvesting time, and warn them against pulling bits of protruding cane from the moving lorries or carts.

In some areas where there are no pavements on the narrow roads and

pedestrians must walk on the road, tell children that it is safer to walk facing the oncoming traffic and in single file.
Make sure children only play with balls in an enclosed space when near a busy road.

REPORTING ACCIDENTS

It must be drilled into the young child starting school that any accident must be reported to an adult. Questions should be asked to discover the exact nature of the accident in the case of a fall when there are no visible external injuries. Attentive observation is needed for any symptoms of illness such as a rise in temperature, listlessness, loss of appetite, that might suggest internal injury.

STRANGERS

Whilst parents do not want to implant a fear of strangers in the young child, they should be told not to accept sweets, fruit or anything from strangers on the street. They must not get into a stranger's car, or be led away by anyone they do not know. It is unfortunate that nowadays in many places a stranger is linked with danger, for in rural areas in many countries children were protected by adults as a general rule. Whilst the majority are still caring adults, every effort must be taken to protect children from those who are not.

Everyone who has responsibility for young children must forever bear in mind the old proverb: 'Prevention is better than cure.'

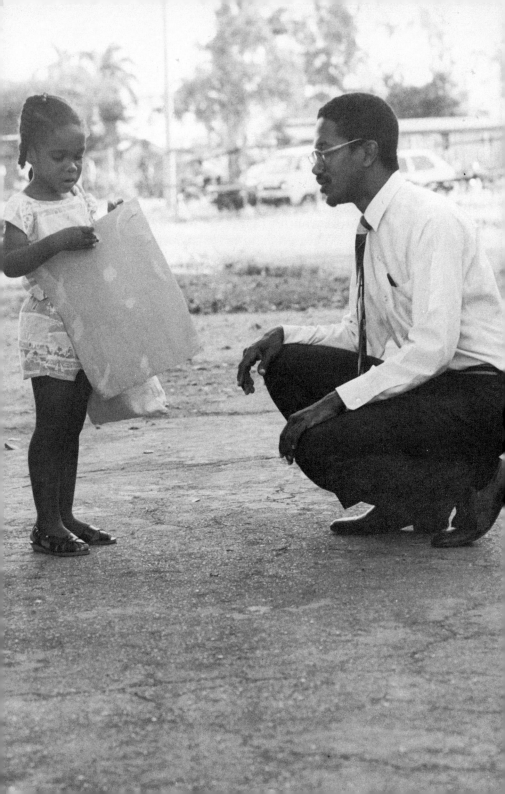

14 The toddler goes to nursery school

In olden days children remained at home learning from the adults around them and helping with the household chores from an early age. Nowadays, since more mothers work outside the home, and because young couples are more likely to live in nuclear families, there is a demand for nursery schools. Nursery schools help to provide a stimulating environment for the toddler and start the preparation for formal education.

SOCIAL DEVELOPMENT

This is very important for the child since it means learning to get along with others. It means learning to wait his turn, to say 'Please' and 'Thank you', to play with others and not to grab the toys he wants. It means learning the meaning of co-operation – for example, in order that the see-saw works properly so that he may enjoy it, he learns that he must go up whilst the other child goes down. Whilst playing, clearing up and putting away the toys and in the daily chats there is opportunity for the exchange of conversation which stimulates verbal development.

EMOTIONAL DEVELOPMENT

From the earliest stages of life, human beings experience love, fear, anger, anxiety, jealousy. At the nursery school the child is helped not only to express feelings but to control them. He learns to direct some of these feelings into purposeful activities. For example, the child who is full of anger, aggressive and likes to fight may be directed to activities which will give him satisfaction, such as playing on the drums, or digging in the garden.

As the child becomes more sure of himself, and begins to achieve more and more, it is observed that anxiety about leaving home lessens and relationships with others begin to be formed.

INTELLECTUAL DEVELOPMENT

The staff at the nursery school ensure that the child develops intellectually. Hand-and-eye co-ordination is developed when letters are looked at and traced; numbers are learnt through rhymes and by seeing them displayed on walls; pouring sand and water from one container to the next teaches the concept of volume and quantities; drawing is preparation for writing; when the teacher reads to him the skills of listening, comprehension and memory are developed, and looking at story books creates familiarity with the printed word.

Some parents worry that after a few months at the nursery school the child is not reading or writing, and feel that the teacher is not 'teaching anything'. If the various methods of learning are explained to parents, they are reassured that the foundation for reading and writing skills are being laid.

MORAL DEVELOPMENT

Children at this stage begin to show a feeling for right and wrong and are quick to tell the teacher who is doing something that is not 'allowed'. This needs to be handled very carefully, as the child should not be encouraged to be a 'tell-tale'.

In some nursery schools where the staff and children are mainly Christian, grace is said at mealtimes, and prayers and hymns are sung. If there are children of other faiths attending, it is not too early to help children to understand and be tolerant of different beliefs.

SEPARATION FROM PARENT

When the toddler leaves home, although only for a few hours, the time will seem very long to be separated from parents and familiar surroundings. At first he may cry and cling to the parent, refusing to be parted from him or her. Most nursery schools allow the parent to stay for some time during the first days until the child settles; a favourite toy or book, if taken along, provides some comfort. Some children may be very insecure and are not sure whether the parent will return. The nursery teacher needs to be patient in introducing the child to the routine of the school.

A normal healthy child is gradually attracted to the brightly coloured toys and play equipment. Seeing other children engaged in activities, he becomes interested, and with a bit of encouragement settles into a routine.

On returning home

When the child returns home he is usually bubbling over with excitement and wanting to show what he has learnt. It is encouraging if parents and other adults in the family show their interest by listening to the stories, rhymes, or songs, asking questions about the activities, and admiring drawings or paintings. These can be displayed on the wall at home by using adhesive tape. It is a good idea to keep the child's work over the years to observe progress, and, later in life, looking back and recalling the early days of school can give a great deal of pleasure to the family.

WEEKENDS AND HOLIDAYS

Because the toddler is interested in everything about him at this age, he needs to be kept occupied. Parents can provide material for him to practise some of the school activities. Sheets of wrapping paper for drawing usually prevent drawing on the wall. Boxes of different sizes will not only give him fun stacking and building but continue the learning experience. This will also help his imagination to develop.

The child may also be allowed to help lay the table, putting out table mats and the cutlery; this provides opportunities for counting and in understanding left and right.

Trips to the market (not during peak hours) are sources of pleasure to a child who lives in urban or suburban areas, as are trips to the countryside to see animals in their natural surroundings.

The toddler also benefits from a quiet time when a parent or other adult reads to him, or sits and encourages looking at pictures and telling stories about them thereby fostering an appreciation of reading; if parents themselves read the child tends to imitate.

At the nursery school the teacher makes sure that the toddler does not become overtired and has a rest period during the day. It is a good idea to continue this practice at home.

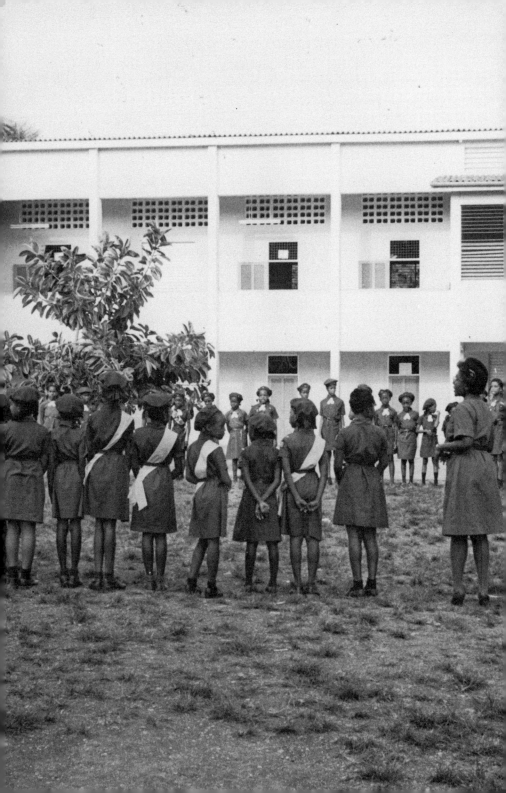

15 Nursery school to infant school

The official age for beginning formal education in schools in most countries is five but some may start at six. By the end of the period in nursery school the average child is ready for what she calls 'big school'.

Most five-year-olds of average intelligence who are well-fed and healthy and grow up in a stable home are eager for the new experience and, if older children in the family attend the same school or one nearby, the move from the informal nursery school to the other is easy. This may not be so for the only child who has stayed at home during the first years, or for the child from an unhappy and unstable home who has been repeatedly told 'You are misbehaving, when you go to school the teacher will beat you if you do not behave.' Very often what is called bad behaviour is the child trying out her growing independence.

THE PHYSICAL CARE OF THE SCHOOL CHILD

The average five-year-old enjoys some self-reliance as certain skills are mastered, such as dressing herself, fastening buttons and snaps, putting shoes on correctly, and likes the opportunity to make choices about her activities. Climbing, skipping, running are frequently selected, but the adult has to make sure that her strength is not over-taxed. The school day is unbroken by a rest period as at nursery school and an early bedtime is advisable as most children of school age still need about 10 or 12 hours' sleep. A sufficient supply of sleep helps to replace the nervous energy used up during the day as well as to supply what is needed for the following day. Where there is television in the home, care needs to be taken that the five- or six-year-old does not sit up to watch until a late hour. Besides the unsuitability of some of the programmes, she loses much-needed sleep. Children who continuously have insufficient sleep are listless, uninterested in the activities around them and slow in learning in the classroom.

THE EARLY YEARS

Food

It helps if the child is wakened in time to eat a well-balanced breakfast which might include milk, eggs, butter bread and fruit. Sometimes, in the excitement of getting off in time, the habit of eating very quickly without properly chewing the food develops. The child who may be reluctant to go to school may eat very slowly and play with the food. Parents need to prevent the first habit from developing by reassuring the child that there is plenty of time, and eating with her to serve as a model. The slow child needs to be dealt with firmly but gently and given small helpings followed by a second helping. She may be given a fruit to take to school to be eaten at breaktime.

In some countries a hot midday meal is provided at school. Some children eat and enjoy the meal, others, especially the slow eater, may not. If the home is near to the school and an adult is at home, it may be possible for the child to go home at midday. Alternatively a packed lunch may be given and a nourishing meal prepared for the evening. If the child is over-tired this also interferes with the appetite and sometimes a rest immediately on getting home helps the child to enjoy the meal better.

Packed lunches

Good packed lunches are balanced, varied and attractively packed. They may consist of: sandwiches with a filling of fish, cheese, egg, or meat; roti with dahl; or spinach cakes. They should also contain a drink made with milk, or a fruit drink and a favourite fruit. Care in the wrapping is necessary so that it is not all soggy and unappetising when opened at lunchtime. This can cause a loss of appetite. The child's diet also plays a part in maintaining good eyesight which is necessary for the increased amount of reading that school entails. Leafy vegetables, carrots, yellow fruits and milk are some of the foods which provide vitamin A, commonly called the 'good eyesight' vitamin.

Personal hygiene

Most families insist on the child being given a bath on mornings before going to school, and hair being combed and brushed, finger nails cleaned and trimmed. This takes time and the child needs to be wakened early so that there is no need to rush or to allow her to go to school in an untidy condition. The child's social development could be hampered by this as other children may shun her.

A bath before going to bed is also very desirable as young children are very active, especially in the playgrounds of schools in the country, where they roll and sit and play on the grass. The child may sometimes object to baths, but parents or other caring adults need to explain the need for the skin to be kept clean so that the pores are not blocked with dirt.

It is advisable to insist on regular and correct brushing of the teeth, especially last thing before going to bed, in order to avoid rapid dental decay.

Frequent brushing and washing of the hair not only makes the child look attractive, but serves to check on whether there is any scalp infection or lice.

When at nursery school there is close supervision of the child after the use of the lavatory, but the same amount of supervision may not be possible at school, so children need to be reminded to wash their hands at school as well as at home.

Constant reminders and repetition of the rules of hygiene are necessary, as the child at this stage is preoccupied with all of the new experiences, and tends to be forgetful.

Clothes

Many schools insist upon children wearing a uniform. One reason for this is that there is no competition between the pupils in the clothes they wear, and a possible source of envy removed. Most parents co-operate with the school even though they may find it a hardship to spend the money on special clothes, but very often they realise that a uniform can be economical.

Well-fitting and roomy underwear which is changed daily helps to keep the child comfortable.

If shoes instead of sandals are worn they need to be well-fitting so as not to interfere with posture. Uncomfortable shoes which cause the feet to hurt are liable to prevent concentration on lessons.

HOME AND SCHOOL

It is essential that the relationship between home and school be a pleasant one. In some rural areas, the parents, who very often know the teacher well, are willing to give full responsibility for the child during school time to the teacher, and expect the teacher to do the best for her. In schools where there are Parent–Teacher Associations the teachers expect the parents to show an interest by attending meetings and to enquire about the progress of their children. The child who knows that parents and teacher communicate is more likely to feel secure that the adults who have responsibility for her welfare are in agreement.

THE CHILD AND THE TEACHER

To the child, the teacher is the source of all knowledge. Very often the family members are told what the teacher says, with emphasis and the conviction that the teacher is right and has the last say. This acceptance of the teacher helps to build the relationship for acceptance of what is taught and helps the progress of the child. It is important that the teachers realise how much influence they have with young children and therefore are prepared to be good models.

Some parents may resent the child's belief in the teacher, believing that their authority is being undermined. They may tell the child 'Never mind what Miss or Sir says.' If this is repeated too often the child can become confused, the loyalties become very divided and it is possible for behaviour problems which interfere with learning to begin.

SOME PROBLEMS OF THE SCHOOL CHILD

Early in the child's school life, the child may well imitate the behaviour of her peers and bring home habits which are not acceptable to the parents, for example, continuous whistling or sitting with feet up on another chair. It should be pointed out that whilst it is good to be friendly one does not always have to follow everything friends do. This is laying the foundation for helping the child to be able to make choices. Fortunately these fashions and fads are not long lasting. Problems which may not have occurred during an earlier stage may surface at this time.

Nail biting

This may begin if new experiences cause anxiety or from imitation of others. Parents should try to discover if it is for emotional reasons and if so try to reassure the child and give her some extra attention. The child should be told of the danger of putting germs and dirt into the mouth. Gentle reminders need to be given to the child rather than shouting 'Do not bite your nails', or slapping. This will increase the anxiety and the habit may continue longer. The little girl's wish to have fingernails like 'Mummy' or her teacher can influence her to stop biting them. The nails should be cut straight across at regular intervals, and the edges filed.

Bedwetting

Most children of school age have become dry at night but may wet the bed occasionally. If this becomes frequent after starting school it may be due to loss of self-confidence in being one among a class in the formal setting of school with a strange teacher. The increased length of the school day may cause overtiredness and sleep is so deep that the child fails to respond to the warning of a full bladder. It could be that the child has developed a fear of the dark and does not get up during the night if she awakens.

Some children do not seem to mind, whilst those who are of a sensitive nature are ashamed or frightened of punishment. The child should not be called dirty or lazy and should not be punished or have threats made to tell friends or teachers. This could make her reluctant to go to school. Some of the following seem to help the child who is physically well, but who continues to wet:

- Avoiding long drinks before going to bed.
- Emptying the bladder immediately before getting into bed.
- Being awakened and taken to the lavatory during the night.
- The use of a potty in the room if she is afraid of the dark.
- Praise when there is a dry bed, reassurance of love and affection, a harmonious atmosphere between the adults in the home.

If the habit continues it is wise to take the child for a thorough physical check.

THE EARLY YEARS

Wetting and soiling clothes

A child may be so timid at school that the teacher's permission to go to the lavatory is not asked and the wetting and soiling of underwear results. It might be helpful if the parent of a shy child reminds her every morning to ask the teacher and also draws the teacher's attention to the problem. If the habit continues in spite of all the efforts made to help the child, it would be advisable for the parent to seek medical advice.

Fears

Depending on the temperament and personality of children, some show more fear than others; also the child may imitate the adults in the family who show fear for various things such as animals, lightning and thunder etc. The child may hear ghost or monster stories at school and develop a fear of the dark. Some adults joke about this fear and frighten the child by making strange sounds or sudden movements if the child enters a dark room. This is not advisable as it can have the effect of deepening the fear. The child needs reassurance from a trusted adult that there is no danger lurking around in the dark. One or other parent may accompany her to bed and remain until she goes to sleep. A dim light may be left in the room and care taken that no objects which cast weird shadows are left in there. The average child learns to control the emotion of fear as she grows up.

Fighting

The child who constantly hits others and frequently fights may be behaving in this way for one of several reasons. Home may be an unhappy place where parents quarrel and fight, where the child is always being punished by flogging, or where an older brother or sister hits her when parents are not around. The new environment of school may be frightening and overpowering, or school work may be difficult and frustrating. Some children stop their aggressive behaviour if they are given opportunities to be responsible such as handing out the pencils in class. Activities which use up the excess energy also help. Talking to the child and giving some extra attention and tuition can go a long way towards making her feel confident about herself.

School refusal

Not all children want to leave mother or the adult who cares for them. In the morning there may be tears or complaints of tummy or headache. As soon as the decision not to send the child to school is reached, a rapid recovery seems to take place. One way of handling this is for the adult to talk it over with the child and so prevent her thinking that the instant recovery went unnoticed. This behaviour may occur if there is a young baby in the family and the school child feels displaced, if a family member goes away or dies, or the parents have separated and the child fears that the other parent may go also. There may be fear of the teacher or of a class bully. Close observation of the child's play and of the conversation with her toys when alone very often gives clues to the cause of the problem. Sometimes assurances from the parent or adult help the child to stop refusing school. The condition worsens the longer she stays at home. The child is not 'bad' and should not be dragged screaming to school, since the refusal is often a symptom of an emotional problem and if it persists, the doctor should be asked to help.

In those countries where psychological services are available the psychologist may discover through the child's play what is upsetting her and is able to advise the parents in ways of handling the problem.

The shy child

The shy and timid child may sit very quietly at school and be reluctant to participate in the activities or to answer when asked a question. Sometimes regressive behaviour such as thumb sucking, bed wetting or stammering may develop. Teacher and parent need to discuss the problem and work together in dealing with the child at home and school in order to build trust and confidence.

The slow child

The slow child who is criticised for being slow and compared unfavourably with others is more likely to develop feelings of uncertainty and believe that 'I can't'. On the other hand when encouragement and patient help are given she has the chance of succeeding to her full capabilities.

PARENTS' INTEREST

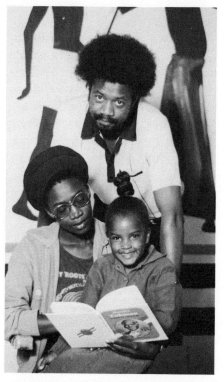

Parents who show interest in the child's activities at school, by talking about them and asking questions, help not only in making the child feel secure, but also in educational development.

There are times when the child needs to be left alone to think, to play quietly and consolidate the many new ideas and experiences of school and the wider environment.

Above all, the example of parents talking to each other, sometimes reading, discussing current topics, listening to the radio or viewing television and taking an interest in the affairs of the community help to give the child a balanced view of living. Praise and encouragement, and opportunities for self-expression also help to build self-confidence.

Children appreciate family life and have definite views about what they would like it to be like. One seven-year-old expresses her view in the following lines:

> It's good to have a mother who will always be there,
> It's good to have a father who will always care,
> It's good to have someone to play with at the lonely times,
> It's good to have a family to care, be there, and keep divine.

Bringing up a child requires time, patience and love. There may be many difficult times. But the joy and excitement of watching her grow and develop into an independent person compensates for any adjustments that have to be made in the parents' living patterns.

Index

accident prevention 157–61
accidents 118, 145–6, 154–7, 161
adoption 27–8
afterbirth 43, 64, 66–7
Aids 39
alcohol during pregnancy 60, 61
antenatal care 51, 52–4, 59, 73
   classes 146, 148
antibiotics 147
artificial respiration 156

bathing the baby 86–90, 95–6, 156
bedwetting 127, 171, 173
behaviour problems 170–3
birth 63, 66, 67
birth-weight of baby 67
   low 68–9
bleeding 145, 156
bottle feeding 76–80
   feeding patterns 80, 95–6
   mixing feeds 77–8
   sterilisation of equipment 77
breastfeeding 23, 67, 68, 69, 73–5, 80, 107–8
   feeding patterns 80, 95–6
breech delivery 66
bowel movements 82, 124
broken bones 156
bruises 154–5
burns and scalds 145, 155
burping the baby 80–1

Caesarean section 65–6
child abuse 19
choking 156
clothing
   during pregnancy 58
   for the baby 90–1, 97
   for the toddler 135
   for the school child 169
colds 145, 150, 151
colic 81
conception 38, 41, 45
contractions 63–5
conjunctivitis 149
contraception *see* family planning
cravings 57
crying
   of baby 85, 96, 97–9, 112
   of toddler 118

development
   pre-natal 41–5

   of baby 23–4, 68, 69, 102–6, 108–9, 115, 129, 132–3
   of toddler 23–4, 109, 125, 133, 163–4
diarrhoea 82, 145
diet
   during pregnancy 55–7, 110
   while breastfeeding 73
   of baby 107–8, 110
   of toddler 113, 120–2, 146
   of school child 168
diphtheria 147, 148
discipline 24, 116–17, 167
divorce 14–15, 18, 26
Down's syndrome 139, 141, 142
drugs during pregnancy 60, 61, 139
dummy 99
dysmenorrhea 36

ear infections 149, 151
ectopic pregnancy 60
embryo 41–3, 60
epidural 65
episiotomy 64
exercise
   during menstruation 36
   during pregnancy 58
   after birth 69
eye infections 148–9

family planning 19, 51, 108
   family planning clinics 21, 39
fears 172
first aid 154, 156
foetus 41–5, 59–60
forceps delivery 65
fostering 28–9, 99

handicapped children 109, 139–43
   causes of handicaps 56, 59, 60
health clinics 21
home confinement 63
hormones 32, 33, 36
hospital confinement 63
hygiene
   during menstruation 35–6
   for children 99, 151–3, 168–9

illness 145–7, 148–51
immunisation 147–8
immunity 74, 145
induction of labour 65
infectious diseases 148–51
infertility 49

INDEX

insect bites 155–6

jealousy of new baby 118, 126–7

labour 63–5
leptospirosis 151

mastoiditis 149
masturbation 125
maternity leave 54
menopause 35
menstrual cycle 33–6
miscarriage 59
'morning sickness' 52
multiple births 48, 49

nail biting 171
nappies
  care of 85
  changing of 82–5
nappy rash 85–6
nausea during pregnancy 52
newborn baby 67–8
  daily routine 95–6
nursery school 112, 113, 125, 127, 145, 163–5, 167, 169

one-parent families 11, 18–19
ovulation 33–4, 41

parenthood 7, 99, 101, 103, 116–17, 119
placenta 41–4, 60
play 101, 108, 118, 129, 131, 134, 135–7, 161, 173
  see also toys
playpen 130
polio 147, 148
post-natal depression 69–70
pregnancy 52–61, 139
  signs of 52
  changes in 22, 51
  duration of 54
premature baby 60, 68–9, 145
pre-menstrual tension 35
punishment 117, 118, 124, 125, 127, 171, 172

registering the birth 70–1
reproductive organs
  female 32–3
  male 36–7
rubella 59, 139

scabies 150, 151
school 167, 170, 173
school child
  problems of 170–3

sex of baby 45–6
sexual intercourse 37
sexually transmitted diseases 38–9
shock 155
shyness 173
sickle cell anaemia 47–8
sleep
  during pregnancy 58
  of new parents 95–6
  of baby 95–7
  of toddler 96, 118–19
  of school child 167
slowness
  to develop 102–3
  at school 173
smoking during pregnancy 60, 61
spina bifida 139, 141
stammering 173
step-parents 26–7, 99
swollen glands 151
syphilis 39

talking
  to the baby 24, 110
  to the toddler 125–6
  to the school child 174
tantrums 123
teeth
  care of during pregnancy 57–8
  of baby 110–12
  care of child's 112–13, 169
teething 111–12
temperature, raised 146, 149, 161
tetanus 147, 148
thumb sucking 122–3, 173
toilet training 124–5
toys 131–4, 159, 165, 173
  for the sick child 147
transporting the baby 92, 93
twins 48–9

ultrasound scan 53
unmarried mothers 14, 70
unplanned pregnancy 19, 101

vomiting
  during pregnancy 52
  of child 81–2, 145, 146, 155

washing the baby 90, 97
  see also bathing the baby
weaning 107–8
wetting and soiling 124, 127, 172
whooping cough 147, 148
working mothers 17–18, 54, 108, 163

X-rays during pregnancy 139